PLAB: 1000 EXTENDED MATCHING QUESTIONS

I dedicate this book to my husband,
William O.A. Coales, MA

PLAB: 1000 EXTENDED MATCHING QUESTIONS

By

Una F. Coales
BA MD FRCS (ED) FRCS (OTO)
Senior House Officer
Department of Otolaryngology
The Royal Surrey County Hospital
Guildford
Surrey, UK

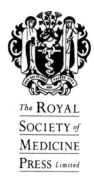

The ROYAL
SOCIETY of
MEDICINE
PRESS Limited

© 2001 Royal Society of Medicine Press Ltd
Reprinted 2001
1 Wimpole Street, London W1G 0AE
207 Westminster Road, Lake Forest IL 60045 USA
www.rsmpress.co.uk

British Library Cataloguing in Publication Data
A catalogue record for this book is available from the British Library

ISBN: 1–85315–472–5

Typeset by Phoenix Photosetting, Chatham, Kent

Printed in Great Britain by Bell and Bain Ltd., Glasgow

Contents

Preface

I was trained in the USA and relocated to the UK to practise surgery. Like many of you readers, I too was faced with the daunting task of how to prepare and to succeed in passing the Professional and Linguistic Assessments Board test (better known as the PLAB exam) to obtain limited registration with the General Medical Council. I passed under the old format.

Since July 2000 the PLAB test has been reformatted. This book is designed to prepare prospective candidates for this new PLAB exam. The format of Part 1 of the PLAB test consists of 200 extended matching questions. To enter Part 2, the candidate must pass Part 1. Part 2 consists of a 14-station objective structured clinical examination (OSCE) and tests your clinical and communication skills.

The 1000 EMQs offered in this book cover all areas stressed by the new PLAB test and are offered in the identical format, testing the four groups of skills required to pass PLAB Part 1. This book also attempts to address all the components of the new syllabus for Part 1 introduced by the General Medical Council. This includes the principles set out in the GMC Publication *Duties of a Doctor*, principles and practice of evidence-based medicine and of clinical governance, questions covering prevalence of important diseases in the UK, risk factors and health promotion.

I would like to thank Miss Philippa Huchzermeyer FRCS (Oto) for editing the questions in otolaryngology, Mr Alak Pal MRCOG for editing the questions in obstetrics and gynaecology, Dr Elizabeth Burrin BSc MBBS for editing the questions in psychiatry, Dr Ashley Smith MRCP for editing the questions in dermatology, and Dr Tim Stewart MBBS for editing the questions in paediatrics.

Don't lose heart, as the PLAB exam is not impossible to pass! Allow me to show you how to tackle the new PLAB test.

Una F. Coales
October 2000

Recommended texts and references

Surgery

Apley A.G. et al (1993) *Apley's System of Orthopaedics and Fractures*, 7th edn.
Arnold, London.

Ellis H. et al (1998) *Lecture Notes on General Surgery*, 9th edn.
Blackwell Scientific Publications, Oxford.

Lattimer C.R. et al (1996) *Key Topics in General Surgery*, 1st edn.
BIOS Scientific Publishers, Oxford.

McLatchie G.R. (1990) *Oxford Handbook of Clinical Surgery*, 1st edn.
Oxford University Press, Oxford.

Unwin A. et al (1995) *Emergency Orthopaedics and Trauma*, 1st edn.
Butterworth-Heinemann, Oxford.

Medicine

Fauci A. et al (1997) *Harrison's Principles of Internal Medicine*, 14th edn.
McGraw-Hill, New York.

Hope R.A. et al (1998) *Oxford Handbook of Clinical Medicine*, 4th edn.
Oxford University Press, Oxford.

Kumar P.J. et al (1998) *Clinical Medicine*, 4th edn.
Baillière Tindall, London.

Rubenstein D. et al (1991) *Lecture Notes on Clinical Medicine*, 5th edn.
Blackwell Scientific Publications, Oxford.

Obstetrics and gynaecology

Chamberlain G. & Hamilton-Fairly D. (1999) *Lecture Notes on Obstetrics & Gynaecology*.
Blackwell Science, Oxford.

Hacker N.F. et al (1998) *Essentials of Obstetrics and Gynaecology*, 3rd edn.
W.B. Saunders Company, Philadelphia.

Paediatrics
Lissauer T. (1996) *Illustrated Textbook of Paediatrics*.
Mosby, London.

Behrman R. et al (1999) *Nelson's Textbook of Pediatrics*.
W.B. Saunders, Philadelphia.

Psychiatry

American Psychiatric Association (2000) *Diagnostic and Statistical Manual of Mental Disorders*, 4th edn. American Psychiatric Association, Washington D.C.

Tomb, D.A. (1999) *Psychiatry*, 6th edn.
Lippincott, Williams and Wilkins, Baltimore.

Otolaryngology

Roland N.J. et al (1995) *Key Topics in Otolaryngology*, 1st edn.
BIOS Scientific Publishers, Oxford.

Question I
Theme: Diagnosis of abdominal pain

Options:

A	Acute appendicitis	J	Pseudo-obstruction
B	Diverticular disease	K	Acute cholecystitis
C	Abdominal aortic aneurysm	L	Acute diverticulitis
D	Perforated peptic ulcer		
E	Crohn's disease		
F	Ulcerative colitis		
G	Acute pancreatitis		
H	Chronic active hepatitis		
I	Acute viral hepatitis		

For each presentation below, choose the SINGLE most likely diagnosis from the above list of options. Each option may be used once, more than once, or not at all.

1. A 20-year-old man presents with colicky periumbilical pain, which shifts to the right iliac fossa, fever, and loss of appetite.

2. A 48-year-old man presents with severe epigastric pain radiating to the back. He is noted to have some bruising in the flanks.

3. A 42-year-old woman presents with anorexia, abdominal pain, and increasing jaundice. She is asthmatic and takes methyldopa for hypertension.

4. A 50-year-old man presents with left-sided colicky iliac fossa pain, change in bowel habits and, rectal bleeding. A thickened mass is palpated in the region of the sigmoid colon. His full blood count is normal.

5. A 78-year-old woman with stable angina presents with massive abdominal distension 10 days following a total hip replacement.

Question 2
Theme: Causes of vaginal discharge

Options:

A	*Trichomonas vaginalis*
B	Gardnerella
C	Chlamydia
D	Gonorrhoea
E	*Mycobacterium tuberculosis*
F	HIV
G	*Lymphogranuloma venerum*
H	*Treponema pallidum*
I	*Granuloma inguinale*

J	*Candida albicans*
K	*Staphylococci aureus*

For each presentation below, choose the SINGLE most likely causative organism from the above list of options. Each option may be used once, more than once, or not at all.

1. A 22-year-old woman presents with intensely irritating yellowish-green frothy vaginal discharge with severe dyspareunia. The organism is seen best under the microscope in a drop of saline.

2. A 30-year-old pregnant woman presents with a thick, white vaginal discharge associated with irritation of the vulva.

3. A 16-year-old girl who uses tampons presents with cervicitis, urethritis, and right knee pain.

4. A 28-year-old woman presents with acute right upper quadrant abdominal pain and watery vaginal discharge. The organism is detected by microimmunofluorescence.

5. A 23-year-old woman presents with fishy smelling vaginal odour. Clue cells are found in the smear.

Question 3
Theme: Investigation of epilepsy

Options:

A	Blood cultures	K	Toxicology
B	Blood glucose	L	Skull X-ray
C	Lumbar puncture		
D	Computed tomography (CT) scan of head		
E	Mantoux test		
F	Electro-encephalogram		
G	Full blood count (FBC)		
H	Chest X-ray		
I	Urea and electrolytes		
J	Blood alcohol level		

For each presentation below, choose the SINGLE most discriminating investigation from the above list of options. Each option may be used once, more than once, or not at all.

1. A 53-year-old obese man presents with sweating, tremor, drowsiness, fits and, agitation. His wife denies any history of alcoholism.

2. A 12-year-old girl is brought to the Accident and Emergency Department by her parents complaining of a persistent rash, photophobia, and neck pain.

3. A 35-year-old mechanic has recurrent epileptiform attacks. He has no history of trauma.

4. An 18-year-old student is brought to the Accident and Emergency Department by ambulance having been flung off his bicycle in a road traffic accident. Upon arrival, he is noted to have deterioration in consciousness.

5. A 32-year-old boxer presents with headache, drowsiness, seizures, and a rising blood pressure.

Question 4
Theme: Causes of vertigo

Options:

A	Meniere's disease	J	Migraine
B	Benign positional vertigo		
C	Acute vestibular neuronitis		
D	Acoustic neuroma		
E	Multiple sclerosis		
F	Iatrogenic vertigo		
G	Cardiovascular disease		
H	Musculoskeletal disease		
I	Hyperventilation		

For each presentation below, choose the SINGLE most likely cause from the above list of options. Each option may be used once, more than once, or not at all.

1. A 42-year-old woman presents with repeated episodes of fluctuating hearing loss, vertigo, and tinnitus lasting hours over the past few months.

2. A 50-year-old man presents with asymmetrical sensorineural hearing loss, dizziness, unilateral tinnitus, and facial pain. He is taking atenolol.

3. A 70-year-old woman presents with vertigo when rolling over in bed. She also notices that she gets dizzy when bending over or reaching for the top shelf.

4. A 56-year-old man complains of dizziness ever since he was a passenger in a car involved in a road traffic accident. His hearing is intact.

5. A 20-year-old anxious woman presents with profound vertigo following an upper respiratory tract infection lasting days.

Question 5
Theme: The treatment of testicular swellings

Options:

A   Surgical exploration of the scrotum
B   Injections of chorionic gonadotrophin
C   Surgical fixation of the testes in the scrotum
D   Orchidectomy alone
E   Orchidectomy followed by radiotherapy
F   Orchidectomy followed by cytotoxic chemotherapy
G   Bedrest and the appropriate antibiotic
H   Surgical removal of the cyst
I   No treatment is required

J   Aspiration of fluid
K   Inguinal herniorraphy

For each case below, choose the SINGLE most appropriate treatment from the above list of options. Each option may be used once, more than once, or not at all.

1. A 14-year-old boy presents with an acutely swollen and painful testis and also pain in the lower abdomen. On examination, the testis lies high in the scrotum.

2. A 35-year-old man presents with a solid testis and abdominal lymph nodes. He has a history of undescended testes as a child.

3. A 20-year-old man presents with a solid testis that is markedly cystic in appearance and lymph node deposits.

4. An 18-year-old man presents with fever, leukocytosis, and a very painful swelling in the testis. Examination of the urine reveals the presence of pus cells.

5. A 60-year-old man presents with a large scrotal swelling that gets in the way of his clothes. On examination, the swelling is fluctuant, and the testis is palpable separately from the swelling.

Question 6
Theme: Principles of the duties of a doctor registered with the General Medical Council

Options:

A   Make the care of your patient your first concern
B   Treat every patient politely and considerately
C   Respect patients' dignity and privacy
D   Listen to patients and respect their views
E   Give patients information in a way they can understand
F   Respect the rights of patients to be fully involved in decisions about their care
G   Keep your professional knowledge and skills up to date
H   Recognise the limits of your professional competence
I   Be honest and trustworthy
J   Respect and protect confidential information
K   Make sure that your personal beliefs do not prejudice your patients' care
L   Act quickly to protect patients from risk if you have good reason to believe that you or a colleague may not be fit to practise
M   Avoid abusing your position as a doctor
N   Work with colleagues in the ways that best serve patients' interests

For each option below, choose the SINGLE most appropriate principle from the list of options. Each option may be used once, more than once, or not at all.

1. A 22-year-old Indian woman requests a female doctor to perform a pelvic exam.

2. A 55-year-old man who is being admitted for a total knee replacement states that he is a Jehovah's witness and therefore refuses any blood products.

3. A 16-year-old girl informs you that she may be pregnant, and her parents are unaware.

4. A 30-year-old man is offered the choice of whether he would like to receive interferon injections for multiple sclerosis.

5. A 60-year-old diabetic sees you for a neurological opinion and asks if you would renew his insulin prescription as a favour.

6. There is a lunch-time teaching session, but a patient on the ward is experiencing chest pain.

7. Your patient reports feelings of depression. You seek a psychiatric opinion.

8. You ask a patient to undress to examine the abdomen. You remember to cover the patient's groin.

9. You are asked to examine a patient at his bedside. You remember to pull the curtain around the bed to ensure privacy.

10. You see an overworked colleague struggle with his duties. You intervene and offer assistance.

Question 7
Theme: Diagnosis of psychiatric disorders

Options:

A   Suicidal risk
B   Alcohol abuse
C   Anxiety
D   Dementia
E   Panic attacks
F   Post-natal problems
G   Opioid abuse
H   Depression
I   Delirium
J   Grief reaction
K   Schizophrenia

For each patient below, choose the SINGLE most likely diagnosis from the above list of options. Each option may be used once, more than once, or not at all.

1. A 70-year-old retired engineer experiences changes in personality and impaired social skills. This is corroborated by his family, who describe him as forgetful and not as sharp. There are no objective features of depression.

2. A 20-year-old man is noted to be withdrawn, isolated, and 'peculiar'. He experiences persecutory delusions and auditory hallucinations.

3. A 60-year-old widow is noted by her family to be restless, disorganised, crying, and frequently expresses her wish to join her deceased partner.

4. A 40-year-old Irishman complains of frequent episodes of chest pains, sweating, palpitations, a sense of impending doom, and trembling that lasts for minutes at a time.

5. A 25-year-old man presents with miosis, slurred speech, disorientation, and respiratory depression.

Question 8
Theme: Diagnosis of childhood illnesses

Options:

A	Measles	J	Pneumococcal meningitis
B	Rubella	K	*Haemophilus influenzae*
C	Varicella zoster		epiglottitis
D	Mumps	L	Streptococcal throat
E	Erythema infectiosum		infection
F	Infectious mononucleosis		
G	Tuberculosis		
H	Typhus		
I	Kawasaki syndrome		

For each patient below, choose the SINGLE most likely diagnosis from the above list of options. Each option may be used once, more than once, or not at all.

1. A 15-year-old girl presents with fever, cough, coryza, and conjunctivitis 9 days after exposure. On examination, she has blue-white punctate lesions on the buccal mucosa.

2. A 17-year-old boy presents with fever, stridor, and trismus. He is noted to be drooling saliva. On examination, he has palpable neck nodes. He fails to respond to a course of penicillin.

3. A 7-year-old girl presents with a low grade fever and a 'slapped cheek', erythematous eruption on her cheeks.

4. A 4-year-old boy presents with an acute onset of fever and a vesicular eruption, following an incubation period of 12 days. The vesicles evolve into pustules and crust over.

5. A 1-year-old baby boy presents with a 5-day history of fever, strawberry tongue, and erythema of the palms and soles. He also has an enlarged 2 cm lymph node.

Question 9
Theme: Causes of dysphagia

Options:

A Achalasia	J Caustic stricture
B Pharyngeal pouch	K Retrosternal goitre
C Diffuse oesophageal spasm	
D Globus pharyngeus	
E Plummer-Vinson syndrome	
F Carcinoma of the oesophagus	
G Peptic stricture	
H Myasthenia gravis	
I Swallowed foreign body	

For each presentation below, choose the SINGLE most likely cause from the above list of options. Each option may be used once, more than once, or not at all.

1. A 32-year-old female presents with progressive dysphagia with regurgitation of fluids. She denies weight loss.

2. A 27-year-old man with a history of depression presents with acute dysphagia. He has a prior history of repeated suicide attempts. There are associated burns in his oropharynx.

3. A 60-year-old woman presents with progressive dysphagia. On exam she has a smooth tongue, koilonychia, and suffers from iron deficiency anaemia.

4. A 65-year-old man presents with regurgitation of food, dysphagia, halitosis, and a sensation of 'lump in the throat'.

5. A 70-year-old man presents with a short history of dysphagia, weight loss, and has palpable neck nodes on examination.

Question 10
Theme: Investigation of weight loss

Options:

A	Stool for cysts, ova and parasites	J	Blood cultures
B	Urea and electrolytes	K	Plasma ACTH and cortisol
C	Chest X-ray		
D	Full blood count		
E	Serum glucose		
F	Urinalysis		
G	Thyroid function tests		
H	Ultrasound of abdomen		
I	Barium swallow		

For each presentation below, choose the SINGLE most discriminating investigation from the above list of options. Each option may be used once, more than once, or not at all.

1. A 60-year-old man recently treated for renal tuberculosis presents with weight loss, diarrhoea, anorexia, hypotension, and is noted to have hyperpigmented buccal mucosa and hand creases.

2. A 50-year-old woman presents with weight loss, increased appetite, sweating, palpitations, preference for cold weather, hot, moist palms, and tremors.

3. A 25-year-old man presents with steatorrhoea, diarrhoea and weight loss after eating contaminated food.

4. A 65-year-old man presents with a sudden onset of diabetes, anorexia, weight loss, epigastric and back pain.

5. A 70-year-old woman presents with progressive dysphagia, weight loss, and a sensation of food sticking in her throat.

Question 11
Theme: Investigation of pyrexia of unknown origin

Options:

A	Haemoglobin	J	Kveim test
B	Full blood count	K	HIV antibody titres
C	Erythrocyte sedimentation rate		
D	Lymph node biopsy		
E	Computerised tomography of the chest		
F	Stool cultures		
G	Mantoux test		
H	Monospot		
I	Echocardiography for vegetations		

For each presentation below, choose the SINGLE most discriminating investigation from the above list of options. Each option may be used once, more than once, or not at all.

1. A 17-year-old boy presents with a 2-week history of fever, malaise, and cervical lymphadenopathy. On examination, he has tenderness in the right upper quadrant of his abdomen and has yellow sclerae.

2. A 25-year-old male drug addict presents with a low-grade fever, malaise, a change in heart murmur, splinter haemorrhages in the nail beds, and Osler's nodes in the finger pulp.

3. A 54-year-old man presents with a 2-month history of unilateral enlargement of his right tonsil, fluctuating pyrexia, and multiple neck nodes.

4. A 25-year-old woman presents with fever, malaise, erythema nodosum, and polyarthralgia. Chest X-ray reveals mediastinal hilar lymphadenopathy.

5. A 29-year-old intravenous drug abuser presents with fever and a neck node discharging a cheesy, malodorous substance.

Question 12
Theme: The treatment of meningitis

Options:

A	Benzylpenicillin	J	Vancomycin
B	Chloramphenicol	K	Supportive
C	Ampicillin		
D	Rifampicin and ethambutol and isoniazid and pyrazinamide		
E	Amphotericin B and flucytosine		
F	Gentamicin		
G	Erythromycin		
H	Cefotaxime		
I	Oral rifampicin		

For each case below, choose the SINGLE most appropriate treatment from the above list of options. Each option may be used once, more than once, or not at all.

1. A 3-year-old girl presents with acute onset of pyrexia, nausea, and vomiting. Lumbar puncture reveals high protein and polymorph count and low glucose. Gram-negative bacilli are present in the smear and culture.

2. A 40-year-old man presents with fever and meningeal signs. His lumbar puncture reveals 20/mm³ mononuclear cells, 2 g/l of protein and a glucose level half his plasma level. There are no organisms in the smear.

3. A 17-year-old girl presents with fever, odd behaviour, purpura, and conjunctival petechiae. Her lumbar puncture reveals gram-negative cocci.

4. A 22-year-old man presents with fever, headache, and drowsiness. His lumbar puncture reveals 1000 mononuclear cells/mm³, 0.5 g/l of protein and a glucose greater than 2/3 of his plasma glucose level. Organisms are absent.

5. The 25-year-old husband of a patient admitted with pyogenic meningitis admits to having oral contact with his wife and is anxious.

Question 13
Theme: Diagnosis of stridor

Options:

A	Laryngomalacia	J	Acute laryngitis
B	Intubation granuloma	K	Multinodular goitre
C	Bilateral recurrent laryngeal nerve palsies		
D	Neck space abscess		
E	Laryngeal papillomatosis		
F	Acute laryngo-tracheo-bronchitis		
G	Subglottic stenosis		
H	Angioneurotic oedema		
I	Acute epiglottitis		

For each patient below, choose the SINGLE most likely diagnosis from the above list of options. Each option may be used once, more than once, or not at all.

1. A 4-year-old girl presents to Casualty with a sudden onset of pyrexia, stridor, and sits with her mouth open and chin forward. She is drooling and in discomfort.

2. A 2-year-old girl presents to Casualty with a week's duration of noisy cough and stridorous breathing. She is lying on her mother's lap.

3. A 40-year-old man presents with fever, stridor, dysphagia, and a neck swelling. He admits to a dental procedure a week prior.

4. A 16-year-old girl presents to Casualty with a rapid onset of stridorous breathing and a petechial rash. She is apyrexial. She is noted to have a swollen uvula and tongue.

5. A 6-month-old baby boy presents to the GP with stridorous breathing. The mother reports that this began a few weeks after birth. His breathing improves when he is lying on his stomach. He is apyrexial. He has always had laboured breathing, worse when feeding.

Question 14
Theme: Causes of infections in pregnancy

Options:

A	Human immunodeficiency virus	J	Cytomegalovirus
B	Gonorrhoea	K	*Toxoplasmosis gondii*
C	Trichomonas		
D	Candidiasis		
E	*Herpes genitalis*		
F	Listeriosis		
G	Rubella		
H	*Treponema pallidum*		
I	Streptococcus		

For each presentation below, choose the SINGLE most likely causative organism from the above list of options. Each option may be used once, more than once, or not at all.

1. A nulliparous woman of 12 weeks gestation presents with diarrhoea, pyrexia, and premature labour. She reports eating unpasteurised cheese and cooked meat.

2. A multiparous woman of 16 weeks gestation reports an intensely itchy, green-coloured, offensive vaginal discharge.

3. A nulliparous woman of 8 weeks gestation is found to have painless ulcers on the labia with regional lymphadenopathy.

4. A nulliparous woman of 10 weeks gestation is found to have shallow painful ulcers on her cervix and labia. She also has associated inguinal lymphadenopathy. She reports recurrent tingling sensation in the affected areas.

5. A nulliparous woman of 12 weeks gestation reports a mild glandular fever-like illness. She has two cats at home.

Question 15
Theme: Diagnosis of abnormal labour

Options:

A	Breech presentation	I	Chorioamnionitis
B	Cephalopelvic disproportion	J	Prolapse of the cord
C	Transverse lie	K	No abnormality
D	Postpartum haemorrhage		
E	Brow presentation		
F	Occipitoposterior position		
G	Preterm premature rupture of membranes		
H	Dysfunctional uterine action		

For each patient below, choose the SINGLE most likely diagnosis from the above list of options. Each option may be used once, more than once, or not at all.

1. A 35-year-old nulliparous woman after prolonged labour delivers twins but has difficulty expelling the placenta. She loses 400 ml of blood vaginally before the placenta is delivered.

2. A 30-year-old multiparous woman of 38 weeks gestation presents with pyrexia, a tender uterus, a foul smelling vaginal discharge, and fetal tachycardia.

3. A 22-year-old primigravid of 36 weeks gestation presents with amniotic fluid coming from the cervix. She is apyrexial.

4. On abdominal exam of a 20-year-old primigravid of 34 weeks gestation, the head of the fetus is found to be in one flank and the buttocks in the other. On vaginal examination, the pelvis is empty of presenting parts. She has a bicornate uterus.

5. A petite 24-year-old primigravid is noted to have a small gynaecoid pelvis and a high head at term. Ultrasound excludes placenta praevia, uterine fibroids, or an ovarian cyst.

Question 16
Theme: Diagnosis of breast diseases

Options:

A	Fibroadenoma		J	Paget's disease
B	Fibrocystic disease		K	Eczema of the nipple
C	Galactocele			
D	Intraductal papilloma			
E	Mammary duct ectasia			
F	Breast cancer			
G	Cystosarcoma phylloides			
H	Breast abscess			
I	Fat necrosis			

For each patient below, choose the SINGLE most likely diagnosis from the above list of options. Each option may be used once, more than once, or not at all.

1. A 28-year-old female presents with a solitary 3 cm freely mobile painless nodule. She also complains of a serous nipple discharge and axillary lymphadenopathy.

2. A 36-year-old female presents with multiple and bilateral cystic breast swellings which are noted to be particularly painful and tender premenstrually. She states that during pregnancy the symptoms improved.

3. A 50-year-old woman presents with nipple discharge, nipple retraction, dilatation of ducts, and chronic intraductal and periductal inflammation. The diagnosis is confirmed by breast biopsy, and no further treatment is required.

4. A 50-year-old woman presents with an eczematoid appearance to her nipple and areola. It is associated with a discrete nodule that is attached to the overlying skin.

5. A 33-year-old lactating female presents with a 1-week history of a painful, erythematous breast lump, and pyrexia. She has tried a course of antibiotics to no avail.

Question 17
Theme: Causes of neck lumps

Options:

A	Branchial cyst	J	Pharyngeal pouch
B	Ludwig's angina	K	Reactive lymphadenitis
C	Parotitis		
D	Thyroglossal cyst		
E	Dermoid cyst		
F	Parapharyngeal abscess		
G	Thyroid swelling		
H	Sialectasis		
I	Laryngocoele		

For each presentation below, choose the SINGLE most likely cause from the above list of options. Each option may be used once, more than once, or not at all.

1. A 45-year-old clarinet player presents with a neck swelling that expands with forced expiration.

2. A 4-year-old boy presents with a small midline neck swelling that moves on swallowing. It is painless, mobile, transilluminates, and fluctuates.

3. A 26-year-old man following a trip to the dentist for a toothache presents with a tender neck swelling, pyrexia, and pain on swallowing. His tonsils are not inflamed.

4. A 30-year-old male presents with a 5 cm neck swelling anterior to the sterno-mastoid muscle on the left side in its upper third. He states that the swelling has been treated with antibiotics for infection in the past.

5. A 20-year-old man presents with a painful swelling under his jaw. On examination, he has trismus and is dribbling saliva.

Question 18
Theme: Causes of anaemia

Options:

A	Vitamin B$_{12}$ deficiency	J	Thalassaemia
B	Iron deficiency	K	Coeliac disease
C	Sickle cell anaemia		
D	Pernicious anaemia		
E	Autoimmune haemolytic anaemia		
F	Hypothyroidism		
G	Sideroblastic anaemia		
H	Anaemia of chronic disease		
I	Glucose-6-phosphate dehydrogenase deficiency		

For each presentation below, choose the SINGLE most likely cause from the above list of options. Each option may be used once, more than once, or not at all.

1. An 8-year-old boy presents with painful swelling of the hands and feet, jaundice, and anaemia. He is noted to have splenomegaly. His blood film has target cells.

2. A 6-month-old baby boy presents with severe anaemia and failure to thrive. His blood film shows target cells, hypo-chromic and microcytic cells. HbF persists.

3. A 40-year-old woman presents with fatigue, dyspnoea, paresthesiae, and a sore, red tongue. Her blood film shows hypersegmented polymorphs, an MCV of > 110 fl, and a low hb.

4. A 60-year-old man post-gastrectomy presents with macrocytic anaemia. He drinks alcohol regularly.

5. A 22-year-old Greek man presents with rapid anaemia and jaundice following treatment of malaria. He is noted to have Heinz bodies.

Question 19
Theme: The treatment of infertility

Options:

    A   In vitro fertilisation
    B   Laparoscopy
    C   Ethinyl oestradiol from days 1 to 10
    D   Salpingolysis
    E   Human menopausal gonadotrophins
    F   Clomiphene citrate
    G   Ligation of varicocoele
    H   Artificial insemination from the husband
    I   Artificial insemination with donor semen

For each case below, choose the SINGLE most appropriate treatment from the above list of options. Each option may be used once, more than once, or not at all.

1. The plasma progesterone level during the luteal phase of the cycle is absent suggestive that ovulation is not occurring. FSH and LH levels are noted to be low.

2. The cervical mucus contact test reveals agglutination of the sperm head-to-head. Sperm antibodies are also noted in the man's plasma.

3. The seminal analysis reveals oligospermia. The husband also suffers from premature ejaculation. The wife has patent tubes and a normal uterus.

4. The post-coital test reveals absence of sperm. The husband has a past history of mumps with orchitis. The wife has patent tubes and a normal uterus.

5. A 35-year-old woman is found to have blocked and severely diseased tubes on laparoscopy. The uterus is normal.

Question 20
Theme: Risk factors for carcinoma

Options:

A	Basal cell carcinoma	J	Breast cancer
B	Oesophageal carcinoma	K	Squamous cell carcinoma of the skin
C	Cancer of the stomach		
D	Bladder carcinoma		
E	Large-bowel carcinoma		
F	Bronchial carcinoma		
G	Nasopharyngeal carcinoma		
H	Oral cancer		
I	Small-bowel tumour		

For each case below, choose the SINGLE most likely type of cancer associated with the risk factors presented. Each option may be used once, more than once, or not at all.

1. A 40-year-old New Zealander presents with an ulcer on the side of his nose. *Rodent BCc*

2. A 55-year-old male smoker has worked in the rubber industry for a decade.

3. A 45-year-old woman with folic acid and iron deficiencies presents with weight loss and bowel habit changes. *coeliac?*

4. A 65-year-old Indian notes a chronic ulcer on his lower lip. He admits to heavy drinking and betel nut chewing.

5. A 70-year-old man admits to asbestos exposure 20 years ago and has attempted to quit smoking. He has noted weight loss and hoarseness of voice.

Question 21
Theme: Diagnosis of fractures

Options:

A	Colles' fracture	J	Bennett's fracture
B	Femoral neck fracture		dislocation
C	Calcaneum fracture	K	Posterior shoulder
D	Scaphoid fracture		dislocation
E	Smith's fracture		
F	Monteggia fracture dislocation		
G	Galeazzi fracture dislocation		
H	Anterior shoulder dislocation		
I	Mallet finger		

For each patient below, choose the SINGLE most likely diagnosis from the above list of options. Each option may be used once, more than once, or not at all.

1. A 27-year-old epileptic man falls onto his outstretched hand and now holds his arm in abduction. The deltoid appears hollow.

2. A 70-year-old female resident of a nursing home is brought into Casualty after falling out of bed. On examination her leg is shortened, adducted and externally rotated. The hip is tender to palpation, and she is unable to weight-bear.

3. A 40-year-old man falls from a tree and lands on his feet. He now presents with painful and swollen heels. His soles are bruised.

4. A 12-year-old presents with a fracture of the lower one third of the radius. She has also sustained a dislocation of the inferior radio-ulnar joint.

5. A 30-year-old cricketer presents with painful phalanx. He cannot actively extend the terminal phalanx of his middle finger.

Question 22
Theme: Investigation of autoimmune disorders

Options:

A	Antinuclear antibody	J	Rheumatoid factor
B	Gastric parietal cell antibody		
C	Smooth muscle antibody		
D	Antibody to mitochondria		
E	Thyroglobulin antibodies		
F	Anti-acetylcholine receptor antibodies		
G	Anti-neutrophil cytoplasmic antibody		
H	Antibody to reticulin		
I	Antibody to platelets		

For each presentation below, choose the SINGLE most discriminating investigation from the above list of options. Each option may be used once, more than once, or not at all.

1. A 44-year-old woman presents with stiff, sausauge-shaped fingers, and MCP joint swelling worse in the morning.

2. A 23-year-old woman presents with diplopia, ptosis, and is unable to count to 50 without her voice tiring. She complains of muscle fatigue.

3. A 20-year-old woman presents with a plethora of signs and symptoms. She complains of arthralgia, depression, alopecia, fits, oral ulceration, and facial rash. She is found to have proteinuria and a normocytic normochromic anaemia.

4. A 40-year-old man presents with a septal perforation, proteinuria, and hypertension.

5. A 50-year-old man presents with vitamin B_{12} deficiency and peripheral neuritis.

Question 23
Theme: Investigation of tumours

Options:

A	Alpha-fetoprotein	K	Cancer antigen (CA-125)
B	Terninal de-oxyribonuclear transferase (TdT)		
C	Carcino-embryonic antigen		
D	Placental alkaline phosphatase		
E	Human chorionic gonadotrophin		
F	Oestrogen receptors (ER)		
G	Squamous cell carcinoma antigen (SCC)		
H	Cancer antigen radio-immunoassay (CA 19.9-RIA)		
I	Calcitonin		
J	Acid phosphatase		

For each presentation below, choose the SINGLE most discriminating tumour marker from the above list of options. Each option may be used once, more than once, or not at all.

1. A 60-year-old man presents with a firm prostate nodule. He is confirmed to have prostate carcinoma on biopsy.

2. A 40-year-old man presents with a thyroid swelling. Fine needle aspirate reveals medullary carcinoma.

3. A 65-year-old man presents with hepatomegaly, weight loss, and jaundice. Abdominal ultrasound reveals hepatic carcinoma.

4. A 23-year-old woman presents with back pain and increasing abdominal girth. She is found to have an epithelial tumour of one ovary.

5. A 35-year-old man presents with an enlarged, smooth, firm testes. He is found to have had a seminoma following orchiectomy.

Question 24
Theme: The treatment of urinary incontinence

Options:

A	Trimethoprim	J	Imipramine
B	Oxybutinin		
C	Ring pessary		
D	Oral hypoglycaemics		
E	Pelvic floor exercises		
F	Vaginal oestrogens		
G	Adjust diuretics		
H	Transurethral resection of the prostate		
I	Laxatives		

For each case below, choose the SINGLE most appropriate treatment from the above list of options. Each option may be used once, more than once, or not at all.

1. A 55-year-old post-menopausal woman complains of urinary incontinence, frequency, and nocturia. The mid-stream urine culture is negative.

2. A 33-year-old woman complains of leaking small amounts of urine when coughing. This began following childbirth.

3. An 80-year-old woman presents with urinary incontinence and is found to have a uterine prolapse. The mid-stream urine culture is negative.

4. A 55-year-old diabetic presents with urge incontinence and an enlarged prostate gland. The mid-stream urine culture is negative.

5. A 50-year-old newly-diagnosed hypertensive complains of urinary frequency and dysuria. The urinanalysis reveals the presence of white cells and protein.

Question 25
Theme: The treatment of postoperative pain

Options:

A	Aspirin tablets
B	Diclofenac suppositories
C	Dihydrocodeine tablets
D	Patient-controlled analgaesia (PCA) with morphine
E	Intercostal nerve blocks
F	Epidural analgaesia
G	Carbamazepine
H	Paracetamol tablets
I	Diamorphine

J   Intramuscular pethidine

For each case below, choose the SINGLE most appropriate treatment from the above list of options. Each option may be used once, more than once, or not at all.

1. A 33-year-old man requires analgaesia following an exploratory laparotomy and splenectomy.

2. A 55-year-old woman with terminal metastatic breast carcinoma requires long-term analgaesia following radical mastectomy.

3. A 40-year-old man complains of phantom limb pain following below-knee amputation.

4. A 25-year-old man underwent excision of a sebaceous cyst under local anaesthesia. He uses salbutamol inhaler on a regular basis.

5. A 60-year-old man requires analgaesia following a total thyroidectomy.

Question 26
Theme: Investigation of postoperative complications

Options:

A   Chest X-ray
B   Serum calcium
C   12-lead electrocardiogram
D   Ultrasound abdomen
E   Serum glucose
F   Mid-stream specimen of urine
G   Thyroid function tests
H   Pulmonary angiogram
I   Bladder ultrasound

J   Serum haemoglobin

For each presentation below, choose the SINGLE most confirmatory investigation from the above list of options. Each option may be used once, more than once, or not at all.

1. A 55-year-old man post thyroidectomy presents with tetany. Upon tapping the preauricular region, the facial muscles begin to twitch.

2. A 50-year-old man post coronary artery bypass graft surgery presents with fever and severe epigastric pain.

3. A 70-year-old woman post dynamic hip screw for a right neck of femur fracture presents with pallor, tachycardia, and hypotension. Her oxygen saturation is 90%. The rest of her examination is normal.

4. A 65-year-old man 10 days post right total hip replacement presents with sudden breathlessness and collapses. On examination, he is noted to have a pleural rub, increased JVP, and a swollen right leg.

5. A 35-year-old primigravida post Caesarian section complains of inability to void. She denies dysuria but complains of fullness. She was treated with an epidural for analgaesia.

Question 27
Theme: Diagnosis of red eye

Options:

A	Acute glaucoma	J	Retinal haemorrhages
B	Iritis		
C	Conjunctivitis		
D	Subconjunctival haemorrhage		
E	Optic neuritis		
F	Conjunctival haemorrhages		
G	Scleritis		
H	Anterior uveitis		
I	Posterior uveitis		

For each patient below, choose the SINGLE most likely diagnosis from the above list of options. Each option may be used once, more than once, or not at all.

1. A 55-year-old woman presents with an entirely red right eye. The iris is injected, and the pupil is fixed and dilated. The intraocular pressure is high.

2. A 20-year-old man presents with a nontender red eye. On examination, the sclera is bright red with a white rim around the limbus. The iris, pupil, cornea, and intraocular pressure are normal.

3. A 33-year-old woman presents with a painful red eye. The conjunctival vessels are injected and blanch on pressure. The iris, pupil, cornea, and intraocular pressures are normal.

4. A 40-year-old man presents with redness most marked around the cornea. The colour does not blanch on pressure. The iris is injected, and the pupil is small and fixed. The cornea and intraocular pressure are normal.

5. A 20-year-old man with nonspecific urethritis and seronegative arthritis is also noted to have red eye associated with Reiter's syndrome.

Question 28
Theme: Diagnosis of skin manifestations of systemic diseases

Options:

A	Erythema nodosum	J	Acanthosis nigricans
B	Erythema multiforme	K	Pretibial muxoedema
C	Erythema marginatum		
D	Erythema chronicum migrans		
E	Vitiligo		
F	Pyoderma gangrenosum		
G	Acquired icthyosis		
H	Necrobiosis lipoidica		
I	Dermatitis herpetiformis		

For each patient below, choose the SINGLE most likely skin manifestation from the above list of options. Each option may be used once, more than once, or not at all.

1. A 53-year-old female presents with proptosis, heat intolerance, and red oedematous swellings over the lateral molleoli which progress to thickened oedema.

2. A 45-year-old man presents with shiny area on his shins with yellowish skin and telangiectasia. He also suffers from areas of fat necrosis.

3. A 55-year-old female who is advised to eat a gluten-free diet presents with itchy blisters in groups on her knees, elbows and scalp.

4. A 30-year-old man suffering from Crohn's disease presents with a pustule on his leg with a tender red-blue necrotic edge.

5. A 15-year-old female presents with fever and mouth ulcers. She is also noted to have target lesions with a central blister on her palms and soles.

Question 29
Theme: Diagnosis of eye problems

Options:

A Flame and blot haemorrhages
B Proliferative retinopathy
C Xanthelasma
D Senile cataracts
E Amaurosis fugax
F Optic atrophy
G Periorbital abscess
H Corneal arcus
I Kayser-Fleischer rings

J Hypertensive fundus
K Lens opacities
L Background retinopathy

For each patient below, choose the SINGLE most likely diagnosis from the above list of options. Each option may be used once, more than once, or not at all.

1. A 65-year-old insulin-dependent diabetic is noted to have a white ring in his cornea surrounding his iris.

2. A 55-year-old man complains of 'a curtain passing over his eyes'. Of note are the presence of carotid bruits on auscultation.

3. A 12-year-old boy, following an episode of sinusitis, complains of persistent pain behind the right eye with eyelid swelling, and diminished vision.

4. A 40-year-old woman complains of pruritis, jaundice, and finger clubbing. She also notes bright yellow plaques on her eyelids.

5. A 30-year-old man is noted to have rubeosis iridis, cotton wool spots, and cluster haemorrhages.

Question 30
Theme: Diagnosis of haematological diseases

Options:

A	Hereditary spherocytosis	J	Acute myeloid leukaemia
B	Myeloid metaplasia	K	Multiple myeloma
C	Uraemia	L	Hodgkin's disease
D	Iron-deficiency anaemia		
E	Sickle cell anaemia		
F	Megaloblastic anaemia		
G	Chronic granulocytic leukaemia		
H	Infectious mononucleosis		
I	Chronic lymphocytic leukaemia		

For each blood smear below, choose the SINGLE most likely diagnosis from the above list of options. Each option may be used once, more than once, or not at all.

1. A 25-year-old female presents with an enlarged, painless lymph node in the neck. She also reports fever and weight loss. Her peripheral blood smear shows Reed-Sternberg cells with a bilobed, mirror-imaged nucleus.

2. A 70-year-old man presents with bone pain, anaemia, and renal failure. His bone marrow reveals an abundance of malignant plasma cells.

3. A 10-year-old boy presents with swelling of the hands and feet and anaemia. His peripheral blood smear reveals target cells and elongated crescent-shaped red blood cells.

4. A 50-year-old insulin-dependent diabetic presents with a 'lemon' tinge to the skin, itching, peripheral oedema, pleural effusions, and anaemia. The peripheral blood smear reveals numerous Burr cells, red blood cells with spiny projections.

5. A 65-year-old woman presents with anaemia. She is noted to have koilonychia and atrophic glossitis. Her blood smear reveals microcytic, hypochromic blood cells.

Question 31
Theme: Causes of bruising

Options:

A	Haemophilia A	J	Christmas disease
B	Side-effect of steroids	K	Henoch-Schonlein purpura
C	Scurvy	L	Leukaemia
D	Idiopathic thrombocytopaenic purpura		
E	Hereditary haemorrhagic telangiectasia		
F	Disseminated intravascular coagulation		
G	Anticoagulant therapy		
H	von Willebrand's disease		
I	Thrombotic thrombocytopaenic purpura		

For each presentation below, choose the SINGLE most likely cause from the above list of options. Each option may be used once, more than once, or not at all.

1. A 10-year-old boy presents with purpura around the buttocks and upper thighs following an upper respiratory tract infection. He also complains of arthralgia and abdominal pain.

2. A 70-year-old man who lives alone presents with ecchymoses of the lower limbs. He has a poor diet lacking fruit and vegetables and suffers from rheumatoid arthritis.

3. A 50-year-old man is noted to have small capillary angiectases on the buccal mucosa and tongue. He has suffered from intermittent gastrointestinal bleeding.

4. A 70-year-old woman presents with epistaxis and bruising. She has a recent history of a deep venous thrombosis.

5. A 20-year-old female presents with fever, abdominal pain, purpura, and focal neurological signs.

Question 32
Theme: The treatment of drug overdoses

Options:

A	Desferrioxamine	J	Dicobalt edetate
B	N-acetylcysteine	K	Hyperbaric oxygen
C	Alkaline diuresis		
D	Naloxone		
E	Supportive therapy only		
F	Diazepam		
G	Flumazenil		
H	Atropine		
I	Phytomenadione		

For each presentation below, choose the SINGLE most appropriate treatment from the above list of options. Each option may be used once, more than once, or not at all.

1. A 70-year-old man presents with severe epistaxis. He is taking warfarin and is noted to have an INR of 8.

2. A 20-year-old presents 8 hours after overdosing on 30 co-proxamol tablets. His stomach is emptied, and further action is needed.

3. A 55-year-old woman presents in respiratory distress after an overdose of diazepam tablets.

4. A 30-year-old primigravida victim of smoke inhalation is brought to Casualty. Her blood gas shows metabolic acidosis, and her COHb is 45%.

5. A 60-year-old hypertensive has overdosed on atenolol by mistake. He now presents with severe bradycardia.

Question 33
Theme: Diagnosis of muscle weakness

Options:

A	Syringomyelia	J	Polymyalgia rheumatica
B	Charcot-Marie Tooth	K	Systemic lupus erythematosus
C	Subacute combined degeneration of the cord		
D	Multiple sclerosis		
E	Bell's palsy		
F	Guillain–Barré syndrome		
G	Poliomyelitis		
H	Motor neurone disease		
I	Dermatomyositis		

For each presentation below, choose the SINGLE most likely diagnosis from the above list of options. Each option may be used once, more than once, or not at all.

1. A 45-year-old woman presents with a purple (heliotrope) rash on her cheeks and eyelids and insidious symmetrical, proximal muscle weakness.

2. A 40-year-old woman presents with diplopia on lateral gaze, nystagmus, paresthesiae, and muscle weakness. CSF from the lumbar puncture reveals oligoclonal bands and an increase in IgG.

3. A 30-year-old man presents a week after an upper respiratory tract infection with paresthesiae which rapidly develops to flaccid paralysis of the lower limbs. The CSF from the lumbar puncture shows very high protein but no white cells.

4. A 25-year-old man presents with flaccid paralysis of the legs with loss of reflexes. He reports recovering from a mild upper respiratory tract infection but then developing meningitis. The CSF shows raised protein and increased lymphocytes.

5. A 35-year-old man presents solely with palsy of the left side of his face including his forehead. His otological exam and other cranial nerves are normal.

Question 34
Theme: Causes of genital tract bleeding in pregnancy

Options:

A Placenta praevia
B Abruptio placenta
C Vasa previa
D Cervical carcinoma
E Ectopic pregnancy
F Cervical polyp
G Vaginal lacerations
H Uterine fibromyomata
I Hydatidiform mole

J Threatened abortion
K Unknown aetiology

For each presentation below, choose the SINGLE most likely diagnosis from the above list of options. Each option may be used once, more than once, or not at all.

1. A 20-year-old nulliparous woman of 30 weeks gestation presents with painless, bright red vaginal bleeding. On ultrasonic examination, the placenta is found to be lying over the internal cervical os.

2. A 44-year-old multiparous woman of 37 weeks gestation presents with heavy dark vaginal bleeding and uterine pain. The uterus is hypertonic and tender to palpation. The fetal lie is longitudinal, and there is an increase in fundal height.

3. A 25-year-old nulliparous woman of 18 weeks gestation presents with uterine pain and mild pyrexia. Pelvic sonogram reveals an enlarged uterus with smoothly rounded protrusions from the uterine wall.

4. A 34-year-old nulliparous woman of 6 weeks gestation presents with painless uterine bleeding. Ultrasound shows no fetal echoes. The hCG levels are high.

5. A 20-year-old nulliparous woman of 8 weeks gestation presents with severe lower abdominal, scant vaginal bleeding, and an empty uterus on ultrasound.

Question 35
Theme: Diagnosis of skin lesions

Options:

A	Lichen planus	J	Dermatitis herpetiformis
B	Psoriasis	K	Pemphigus vulgaris
C	Pityriasis versicolor	L	Pemphigoid
D	Pityriasis rosea		
E	Acne vulgaris		
F	Allergic contact dermatitis		
G	Acanthosis nigricans		
H	Herpes zoster		
I	Erythema nodosum		

For each presentation below, choose the SINGLE most likely diagnosis from the above list of options. Each option may be used once, more than once, or not at all.

1. A 80-year-old man presents with itching followed by large, tense bullae on the limbs that do not rupture easily. Nikolsky's sign is negative.

2. A 50-year-old man presents with brownish scaly lesions of varying sizes on his trunk. Depigmentation after treatment lasts for several months.

3. A 30-year-old female presents with an itchy painful rash over the lobes of both pinna. Her earlobes are pierced.

4. A 50-year-old man presents with a rash consisting of discrete purple shiny polygonal papules with fine white lines in previous scratch marks on his forearm. He is also noted to have a white lacy network of lesions on the buccal mucosa.

5. A 60-year-old man presents with brown pigmented plaques in the axilla. He underwent prostatectomy recently.

Question 36
Theme: Diagnosis of heart conditions

Options:

A   Anterolateral myocardial   J   Aortic regurgitation
     infarction   K   Inferolateral myocardiol
B   Left ventricular failure   infarction
C   Atrial fibrillation
D   Acute pulmonary embolism
E   Acute pericarditis
F   Mitral stenosis
G   Right ventricular failure
H   Hypokalaemia
I   Hypocalcaemia

For each presentation below, choose the SINGLE most likely diagnosis from the above list of options. Each option may be used once, more than once, or not at all.

1. A 60-year-old man presents with chest pain radiating down the left arm. His 12-lead electrocardiogram reveals Q waves in II, III and AVf with T wave changes in V5 and V6.

2. A 50-year-old woman presents with a fast heart rate with an irregular rhythm. There are no P waves on the electrocardiogram. She states that she has lost weight recently and is 'nervous'. She also suffers from palpitations.

3. On auscultation, a patient is noted to have a rumbling diastolic murmur at the apex. The murmur is accentuated during exercise.

4. A 60-year-old man on digitalis and diuretics presents with weakness and lethargy. His electrocardiogram shows flat T waves and prominent U waves.

5. A 65-year-old man with chronic bronchitis presents with a raised jugular venous pressure, hepatomegaly, ankle and sacral oedema.

Question 37
Theme: Investigation of collapse

Options:

A	Blood glucose	J	Ultrasound abdomen
B	Full blood count	K	Urine pregnancy test
C	Computed tomography scan of the head		
D	Electrocardiogram		
E	Chest X-ray		
F	Lumbar puncture		
G	Urea and electrolytes		
H	Pelvic ultrasound		
I	Thyroid function tests		

For each presentation below, choose the SINGLE most discriminating investigation from the above list of options. Each option may be used once, more than once, or not at all.

1. A 20-year-old college student presents to the Accident and Emergency Department after collapsing at school. Her last menstrual period was 3 weeks ago and lasted 3 days. She is anxious. Her pulse is irregular and rapid.

2. A 16-year-old girl is brought in to her GP after collapsing. She is noted to be febrile with a purpuric rash that does not blanch on pressure.

3. A 22-year-old female presents to her GP after collapsing at home. She reports nausea worse in the morning. Her last menstrual period was 5 weeks ago.

4. A 60-year-old female is brought into the Accident and Emergency Department after collapsing at home. Her thighs show evidence of lipoatrophy and her shins of necrobiosis lipoidica.

5. A 30-year-old man presents to Casualty after collapsing on the cricket pitch. He takes carbamazepine. There is a haematoma over his right temple.

Question 38
Theme: Investigation of abdominal pain

Options:

A	Ultrasound abdomen	J	Laparoscopy
B	Rectal examination	K	Erect chest X-ray
C	Upper GI endoscopy		
D	Barium meal		
E	Sigmoidoscopy		
F	Colonoscopy		
G	Computed tomography scan of the abdomen		
H	Kidneys, ureters and bladder (KUB) X-ray		
I	Pelvic ultrasound		

For each presentation below, choose the SINGLE most discriminating investigation from the above list of options. Each option may be used once, more than once, or not at all.

1. A 60-year-old man complains of severe colicky pain from his right flank radiating to his groin. His urinalysis reveals trace blood cells.

2. A 25-year-old woman complains of severe lower abdominal pain and increasing abdominal girth. Her urine HCG is negative.

3. A 60-year-old obese man complains of severe epigastric pain radiating to his back. The pain is relieved by eating and is worse at night.

4. A 65-year-old hypertensive man presents with lower abdominal pain and back pain. An expansive abdominal mass is palpated lateral and superior to the umbilicus.

5. An 80-year-old woman suffering from rheumatoid arthritis presents with severe epigastric pain and vomiting. She also complains of shoulder tip pain.

Question 39
Theme: Diagnosis of childhood extremity pain

Options:

A	Non-accidental injury	J	Growing pains
B	Chondromalacia patella	K	Systemic lupus
C	Slipped femoral epiphysis		erythematosus
D	Osgood-Schlatter disease		
E	Sickle cell disease		
F	Juvenile rheumatoid arthritis		
G	Influenza		
H	Reactive arthritis		
I	Transient synovitis of the hip		

For each case below, choose the SINGLE most likely diagnosis from the above list of options. Each option may be used once, more than once, or not at all.

1. A 15-year-old female presents with fever, arthritis, weight loss, and fatigue. Urinalysis reveals protein, red blood cells, and casts. Lab results reveal the presence of antinuclear antibodies and antibodies to double-stranded DNA.

2. A 4-year-old girl presents with a 2-month history of arthritis involving the knees and ankles. She is noted to have irido-cyclitis on slit lamp examination. The ANA is positive, and the rheumatoid factor is negative.

3. An 8-year-old girl presents with recurrent extremity pain. On exam she is found to have yellow-green bruises on her calf and a 1 cm circular scar on her palm.

4. A 15-year-old boy presents with a limp and pain in the knee. On clinical examination, the leg is externally rotated and 2 cm shorter. There is limitation of flexion, abduction, and medial rotation. As the hip is flexed, external rotation is increased.

5. A 13-year-old girl presents with a painful and swollen knee. There is no history of injury. A tender lump is palpated over the tibial tuberosity.

Question 40
Theme: The treatment of skin conditions

Options:

A   Topical coal tar
B   Topical steroids
C   Clotrimazole
D   Erythromycin
E   Adrenaline
F   Oral prednisolone
G   Dapsone
H   Oxytetracycline
I   Cetrimide
J   Acyclovir
K   Oral nystatin

For each case below, choose the SINGLE most appropriate treatment from the above list of options. Each option may be used once, more than once, or not at all.

1. A 24-year-old man presents with multiple silver-scaly lesions over the extensor surfaces of his elbows and knees. He also has nail pitting and arthropathy of the terminal interphalangeal joints.

2. An 18-year-old female presents with an itchy rash along the flexor surfaces of her elbows and knees. Scaling and weeping vesicles are features.

3. A 23-year-old female with Hodgkin's disease presents with small, white mucosal flecks in the mouth that can be wiped off.

4. A 50-year-old man presents with flaccid bullae over the limbs and trunk following a course of penicillamine for his rheumatoid arthritis.

5. A 20-year-old hairdresser presents with itchy vesicles on her palms.

Question 41
Theme: Causes of hypertension

Options:

A	Coarctation of the aorta	J	Renal artery stenosis
B	Cushing's syndrome	K	Chronic glomerulo-
C	Pheochromocytoma		nephritis
D	Primary hyperaldosteronism		
E	Polyarteritis nodosa		
F	Polycystic kidneys		
G	Acromegaly		
H	Pre-eclampsia		
I	Essential hypertension		

For each presentation below, choose the SINGLE most likely cause from the above list of options. Each option may be used once, more than once, or not at all.

1. A 45-year-old woman presents with hypertension and confusion. She is noted to have truncal obesity, proximal myopathy, and osteoporosis. She has a raised 24-hour urinary free cortisol level.

2. A 35-year-old man presents with hypertension and complains of tingling in his fingers. He is noted to have an enlarged tongue and prognathism. His glucose tolerance curve is diabetic.

3. A 45-year-old woman with disproportionately long limbs presents with hypertension. Her blood pressure is different on both arms and lower in the legs.

4. A 40-year-old man post thyroidectomy for medullary thyroid carcinoma presents with hypertension and complains of attacks of severe headache and palpitations. He is noted to have glycosuria.

5. A 50-year-old man presents with hypertension, haematuria, and abdominal pain. A large kidney is palpated on exam, and the diagnosis is confirmed on ultrasound.

Question 42
Theme: Causes of peripheral neuropathy

Options:

A	Carcinomatous neuropathy	J	Industrial poisoning
B	Side-effect of drug therapy	K	Porphyria
C	Diabetic neuropathy		
D	Vitamin B_{12} deficiency		
E	Vitamin B_1 deficiency		
F	Polyarteritis nodosa		
G	Guillain–Barré syndrome		
H	Amyloidosis		
I	Sarcoidosis		

For each patient below, choose the SINGLE most likely diagnosis from the above list of options. Each option may be used once, more than once, or not at all.

1. A 50-year-old man presents with distal sensory neuropathy affecting the lower limbs in a 'stocking' distribution and is noted to have Charcot's joints. The ankle reflex is absent.

2. A 55-year-old man who drinks heavily presents with numbness and paresthesiae in his feet. He complains of 'walking on cotton wool'.

3. A 40-year-old man, who is being treated with chemotherapy for lymphoma, presents with peripheral paresthesiae, loss of deep tendon reflexes, and abdominal bloating.

4. A 45-year-old woman presents with peripheral neuropathy. She is noted to have bilateral hilar gland enlargement on chest X-ray and a negative Mantoux test. She also suffers from polyarthralgia and has tender red, raised lesions on her shin.

5. A 25-year-old man presents with paresthesiae followed by a flaccid paralysis of his limbs and face. He has a history of a recent upper respiratory tract infection.

Question 43
Theme: Diagnosis of pulmonary diseases

Options:

A	Pneumoconiosis
B	Cystic fibrosis
C	Mycoplasma pneumonia
D	Adult respiratory distress syndrome
E	Pulmonary contusion
F	Carcinoma of the bronchus
G	Pancoast's tumour
H	Bilateral bronchopneumonia
I	Sarcoidosis

J   Tuberculosis

For each case below, choose the SINGLE most likely diagnosis from the above list of options. Each option may be used once, more than once, or not at all.

1. A 30-year-old woman presents with fever, pharyngitis, and cough. The chest X-ray shows widespread, bilateral, patchy consolidation. Cold agglutinins are detected.

2. A 40-year-old alcoholic presents with repeated small haemoptysis and cough with mucoid sputum. His chest X-ray shows right upper lobe consolidation and a large central cavity. His Heaf test is positive.

3. A 60-year-old man presents with dyspnoea and cough. The X-ray shows extensive pulmonary fibrosis, bilateral pleural thickening, and pleural calcification.

4. A 14-year-old boy presents with repeated lower respiratory infections. On examination he is noted to have finger clubbing and suffers from weight loss and steatorrhoea. The X-ray shows bronchial wall thickening, ring shadows of bronchiectasis, and wide-spread ill-defined shadowing.

5. A 40-year-old man presents with cough and haemoptysis. The X-ray shows a right hilar mass and a patch of consolidation in the right upper lobe laterally.

Question 44
Theme: Investigation of weight problems

Options:

A Ultrasound abdomen
B Thyroid function tests
C Short ACTH stimulation test
D Chest X-ray
E Upper GI endoscopy
F Blood glucose
G 24 hour urine collection for vanillyl-mandelic acid
H Proctosigmoidoscopy
I 24 hour collection for urine-free cortisol
J Stool culture

For each presentation below, choose the SINGLE most discriminating investigation from the above list of options. Each option may be used once, more than once, or not at all.

1. A 20-year-old man presents with intermittent abdominal pain with diarrhoea and weight loss. He is noted to have anal lesions, clubbing, arthritis, and erythema nodosum.

2. A 40-year-old woman presents with weight gain and truncal obesity. She suffers from amenorrhoea, hirsuitism, hypertension, and is noted to have glycosuria.

3. A 30-year-old insulin-dependent diabetic presents with weight loss, weakness, vitiligo, and hyperpigmentation of the palmar creases. His serum electrolytes are abnormal.

4. A 20-year-old female presents with an insidious onset of weight gain, hoarseness, and menorrhagia. Her mother states that she is depressed of late.

5. A 15-year-old girl presents with a few weeks history of weight loss, polyuria, and polydipsia.

Question 45
Theme: The treatment of hypertension

Options:

A	Atenolol	J	Lisinopril
B	Bendrofluazide	K	Non-drug treatment
C	Frusemide		
D	Methyldopa		
E	Amlodipine		
F	Nifedipine		
G	Hydralazine		
H	Captopril		
I	Sodium nitroprusside		

For each patient below, choose the SINGLE most appropriate treatment from the above list of options. Each option may be used once, more than once, or not at all.

1. A 60-year-old man presents with a BP of 165/95. He is asymptomatic, and all his investigations are normal.

2. A 55-year-old insulin-dependent diabetic presents to his GP with a BP of 170/110. His blood pressure is consistently high on subsequent visits despite conservative measures. His blood tests are normal.

3. A 50-year-old asthmatic presents to his GP with a BP of 180/120. All underlying causes have been excluded.

4. A 60-year-old man is brought into Accident and Emergency complaining of severe headaches. On arrival he has a seizure. His BP is noted to be 220/140, and on fundoscopic exam, there is papilloedema.

5. A 66-year-old man on atenolol 100 mg od continues to have a diastolic blood pressure of 115. He also takes allopurinol. A second drug is recommended.

Question 46
Theme: The treatment of respiratory diseases

Options:

A	Erythromycin	J	Salbutamol inhaler
B	Tetracycline	K	Ciprofloxacin
C	Flucloxacillin		
D	Benzylpenicillin		
E	Cefotaxime		
F	Prednisolone		
G	Rifampicin, isoniazid, pyridoxine and ethambutol		
H	Isoniazid alone		
I	Cotrimoxazole		

For each case below, choose the SINGLE most appropriate treatment from the above list of options. Each option may be used once, more than once, or not at all.

1. A 20-year-old woman presents with a week's history of fever, rigors, and productive, rusty cough. The X-ray shows a left lower lobe consolidation.

2. A 12-year-old boy with cystic fibrosis presents with a persistent productive cough. The X-ray shows a spherical shadow containing a central lucency. An air-fluid level is also seen.

3. A 50-year-old man presents with shortness of breath and dry cough. The X-ray shows wide-spread pulmonary shadowing. He takes azathioprine for resistant rheumatoid arthritis.

4. A 20-year-old female presents with malaise, cough and progressive shortness of breath. The X-ray shows symmetrical lobulated bilateral hilar gland enlargement.

5. A 50-year-old diabetic presents with a productive cough and malaise. The X-ray shows right upper lobe consolidation and hilar lymphadenopathy.

Question 47
Theme: Diagnosis of hearing problems

Options:

A	Presbyacusis	I	Otosclerosis
B	Cerumen	J	Temporal bone fracture
C	Acute suppurative otitis media	K	Osteogenesis imperfecta
D	Otitis externa		
E	Chronic secretory otitis media		
F	Barotrauma		
G	Chronic suppurative otitis media		
H	Dead ear		

For each patient below, choose the SINGLE most likely diagnosis from the above list of options. Each option may be used once, more than once, or not at all.

1. A 70-year-old man presents with gradual deterioration of hearing in both ears. His Weber tuning fork test is nonlateralising, and his Rinne test is positive on both sides. His tympanic membranes are intact and healthy.

2. A 60-year-old man presents with unilateral earache, diminished hearing, and foul-smelling discharge. The external auditory meatus is oedematous, and the canal is stenosed. The discharge is white and creamy in nature.

3. A 40-year-old woman presents with diminished hearing in the right ear. She denies earache or discharge. She is noted to have blue sclerae. The tympanic membrane is normal. The Weber tuning fork test lateralises to the right side, and the Rinne is negative on the right.

4. A 4-year-old girl presents to her GP with diminished hearing noted by the school. On examination, she has a bulging yellow tympanic membrane on the right alone.

5. A 70-year-old female presents with longstanding deafness in the left ear. The Weber lateralises to the right, and the Rinne is negative on the left.

Question 48
Theme: Diagnosis of jaundice

Options:

A	Cholestatic jaundice	J	Primary biliary cirrhosis
B	Hepatitis A		
C	Haemolytic jaundice		
D	Crigler-Najjar syndrome		
E	Gilbert's syndrome		
F	Chronic active hepatitis		
G	Hepatitis B		
H	Alcoholic hepatitis		
I	Leptospirosis		

For each patient below, choose the SINGLE most likely diagnosis from the above list of options. Each option may be used once, more than once, or not at all.

1. A 35-year-old IVDA on penicillin and flucloxacillin for cellulitis now presents with jaundice, pale stools, and dark urine.

2. A 20-year-old man presents with mild jaundice following an upper respiratory tract infection. On fasting, his bilirubin level is high.

3. A 20-year-old woman presents with abdominal pain, increasing jaundice, and arthralgia. She is noted to have hepatosplenomegaly. She recently donated blood. She is found to have an increase in both conjugated and unconjugated bilirubin.

4. A 45-year-old woman presents with pruritis, jaundice and pigmentation. Both the liver and spleen are palpable. Investigations reveal a high alkaline phosphatase and a high bilirubin.

5. A 55-year-old man presents with pale stool and jaundice. Three days earlier he had fever, malaise, vomiting, and upper abdominal discomfort associated with tender enlargement of the liver. He takes methyldopa for hypertension.

Question 49
Theme: Causes of arthritis

Options:

A	Gout	J	Haemochromatosis
B	Rheumatoid arthritis	K	Gonococcal arthritis
C	Psoriatic arthropathy		
D	Pyrophosphate arthropathy		
E	Ankylosing spondylitis		
F	Reiter's syndrome		
G	Systemic lupus erythematosus		
H	Hyperparathyroidism		
I	Osteoarthritis		

For each patient below, choose the SINGLE most likely cause from the above list of options. Each option may be used once, more than once, or not at all.

1. A 20-year-old man presents with urethritis and a swollen painful wrist.

2. A 25-year-old man presents with urethritis, conjunctivitis, and a swollen left knee.

3. A 50-year-old woman complains of stiffness in her fingers worse at the end of the day. The DIP joints and the first metacarpophalangeal joints are affected.

4. A 20-year-old man presents with morning stiffness, sacroiliitis, and iritis.

5. A 22-year-old man presents with a red, hot, swollen metatarsal phalangeal joint, sacroiliitis, and onycholysis.

Question 50
Theme: Investigation of vomiting

Options:

A	Full blood count (FBC)	J	Blood glucose
B	Erect chest X-ray	K	Mid-stream specimen of urine
C	Plasma cortisol level		
D	Computed tomography (CT) scan of head		
E	Serum calcium		
F	Urea and electrolytes		
G	Ultrasound abdomen		
H	Urinary phorphobilinogen (PBG) and d-amino-laevulinic (ALA)-synthetase		
I	Thyroid function tests		

For each presentation below, choose the SINGLE most discriminating investigation from the above list of options. Each option may be used once, more than once, or not at all.

1. A 60-year-old man on insulin presents with itching, nausea, and vomiting. He is noted to have peripheral oedema and normocytic anaemia.

2. A 50-year-old woman with known breast carcinoma presents acutely with nausea, vomiting, polydypsia, confusion, and drowsiness.

3. A 30-year-old woman with Hodgkin's disease presents with an insidious onset of weakness, weight loss, nausea, and vomiting. She is noted to have hyperpigmented hand creases.

4. A 30-year-old woman started on oral contraceptives presents acutely with abdominal pain, vomiting, tachycardia, hypertension and peripheral neuropathy.

5. A 30-year-old man involved in a RTA presents acutely with severe epigastric pain, left shoulder pain, and vomiting. He has no bowel sounds.

Question 51
Theme: Diagnosis of abdominal pain in pregnancy

Options:

A	Peptic ulcer disease		J	Abruptio placentae
B	Fulminating pre-eclampsia		K	Hydramnios
C	Appendicitis		L	Pyelonephritis
D	Abortion			
E	Fibroids			
F	Cholecystitis			
G	Ectopic pregnancy			
H	Urinary infection			
I	Ureteric stone			

For each patient below, choose the SINGLE most likely diagnosis from the above list of options. Each option may be used once, more than once, or not at all.

1. A 33-year-old multiparous woman of 32 weeks gestation complains of severe back pain. The urinanalysis reveals red blood cells. She is apyrexial.

2. A 25-year-old primigravid of 8 weeks gestation presents with severe lower abdominal cramping, vaginal bleeding, and the passage of clots. The internal os is open.

3. A 28-year-old primigravid of 10 weeks gestation presents with sudden, severe lower abdominal pain. Her abdomen is rigid and the uterus tender.

4. A 30-year-old multiparous woman of 12 weeks gestation presents with lower abdominal pain and tenderness. She also complains of urinary frequency. She is apyrexial.

5. A 26-year-old nulliparous woman of 20 weeks gestation presents with headache and epigastric pain. Her BP is noted to be 150/100 and rising.

Question 52
Theme: The treament of coma

Options:

A	Cefotaxime IV	J	Benzylpenicillin IV
B	Phentolamine IV	K	Acyclovir IV
C	Triiodothyronine IV		
D	Propranolol IV		
E	Insulin infusion		
F	50% dextrose IV		
G	Neurosurgical decompression dependent on CT scan findings		
H	Naloxone IV		
I	Hydrocortisone sodium succinate IV		

For each case below, choose the SINGLE most appropriate treatment from the above list of options. Each option may be used once, more than once, or not at all.

1. A 22-year-old man involved in a RTA presents to Accident and Emergency comatose with pinpoint pupils.

2. A 30-year-old man with a history of epilepsy is brought to Accident and Emergency in a comatose state. He is pyrexial and noted to have a purpuric rash. His family states that he is allergic to penicillin.

3. A 55-year-old man undergoing an intravenous urogram suddenly complains of severe headache and palpitations. His BP is noted to be 180/120 and rising.

4. A 50-year-old man is brought into Accident and Emergency in a comatose state. He smells of alcohol. He is apyrexial with a BP of 180/110 and a pulse of 50. His pupils are unequal.

5. A 70-year-old man is brought to Accident and Emergency in a coma. His temperature is 35°C, pulse is 50, and he has a goitre on exam.

Question 53
Theme: Causes of pneumonia

Options:

A   *Chlamydia psittaci*   J   *Pseudomonas aeruginosa*
B   *Pneumocystis carinii*   K   *Legionalla pneumophilia*
C   *Mycoplasma pneumoniae*
D   Tuberculosis
E   *Coxiella burnetii*
F   Aspergillosis
G   Actinomycosis
H   *Streptococcus pneumoniae*
I   *Staphylococcus aureus*

For each presentation below, choose the SINGLE most likely causative organism from the above list of options. Each option may be used once, more than once, or not at all.

1. A 35-year-old pet-shop owner presents with high fever, excruciating headache, and a dry hacking cough. The X-ray shows patchy consolidation.

2. A 40-year-old man who works in an abattoir presents with a sudden onset of fever, myalgia, headache, dry cough, and chest pain. The X-ray shows patchy consolidation of the right lower lobe, giving a ground-glass appearance.

3. A 44-year-old travelling insurance salesman presents with high fever, myalgia, abdominal pain, and haemoptysis. The X-ray shows diffuse, patchy, lobar shadows. The cough progresses from a modest nonproductive cough to producing muco-purulent sputum. The fever persists for 2 weeks.

4. A 30-year-old man with HIV presents with a productive cough and haemoptysis. The X-ray shows a round ball in the right upper lobe surmounted by a dome of air.

5. A 70-year-old woman presents with confusion and productive cough. The X-ray shows right lower lobe consolidation.

Options:

A	Ischaemic ulcer	J	Aphthous ulcers
B	Basal cell carcinoma		
C	Squamous cell carcinoma		
D	Syphilis		
E	Tuberculosis		
F	Trophic ulcer		
G	Venous ulcer		
H	Barrett's ulcer		
I	Behçet's disease		

For each patient below, choose the SINGLE most likely diagnosis from the above list of options. Each option may be used once, more than once, or not at all.

1. A 60-year-old man presents with a superficial leg ulcer. The ulcer has a sloping edge, and the skin around the edge is red-blue and almost transparent.

2. A 70-year-old man presents with an ulcer on the right pinna with palpable neck nodes. The edges of the ulcer are everted.

3. A 50-year-old man presents with an ulcer on the left side of his nose. The edges are rolled.

4. A 60-year-old man presents with painful ulcers in the oral mucosa. He underwent cholecystectomy a week prior. The edges are erythematous.

5. A 30-year-old woman presents with painful ulcers of the labia and mouth. She also suffers from arthritis.

Question 55
Theme: Causes of splenomegaly

Options:

A	Typhoid		J	Leptospirosis
B	Gaucher's disease		K	Chronic myeloid
C	Malaria			leukaemia
D	Schistosomiasis			
E	Lymphoma			
F	Leishmaniasis			
G	Idiopathic thrombocytopaenic purpura			
H	Polycythaemia rubra vera			
I	Felty's syndrome			

For each case below, choose the SINGLE most likely cause from the above list of options. Each option may be used once, more than once, or not at all.

1. A 20-year-old man presents acutely with fever, jaundice, purpura, injected conjunctiva, and painful calves after swimming outdoors.

2. A 26-year-old man recently returned from a trip to India presents with intermittent fevers, cough, diarrhoea, epistaxis and massive splenomegaly.

3. A 22-year-old female presents with epistaxis and easy bruising. Her spleen is noted to be enlarged.

4. A 30-year-old Jewish man presents with incidental splenomegaly on a routine physical exam at his GP's clinic. His serum acid phosphatase is elevated. He admits to having episodes of bone pain. His uncle also has an enlarged spleen.

5. A 60-year-old female with rheumatoid arthritis presents with splenomegaly. Her full blood count shows a white count of 1500/mm^3.

Options:

A	Volkmann's ischaemic contracture	J	Koilonychia
		K	Glomus tumour
B	Dupuytren's contracture	L	Subungual haematoma
C	Carpal tunnel syndrome		
D	Claw hand		
E	Raynaud's phenomenon		
F	Scleroderma		
G	Rheumatoid arthritis		
H	Paronychia		
I	Psoriasis		

For each presentation below, choose the SINGLE most likely diagnosis from the above list of options. Each option may be used once, more than once, or not at all.

1. A 20-year-old female presents with a painful fingertip that throbs and has kept the patient up all night. The skin at the base and side of the nail is red, tender, and bulging.

2. A 30-year-old female presents with a painful fingernail. On examination, there is a small purple-red spot beneath the nail. She denies trauma to the finger.

3. A 60-year-old man with acromegaly presents with pins and needles in the index and middle fingers of his right hand, worse at night.

4. A 20-year-old man presents with fingers that are permanently flexed in his right hand. However, the deformity is abolished by flexion of the wrist. He admits to trauma to his elbow recently. He also complains of pins and needles.

5. A 20-year-old female complains of intermittent pain in her fingertips. She describes the fingers undergoing colour changes from white to blue and then to red. The symptoms are worse in the winter.

Question 57
Theme: Causes of haematuria

Options:

A	Ureteric calculus	J	Renal vein thrombosis
B	Acute pyelonephritis	K	Acute intermittent
C	Benign prostatic hypertrophy		porphyria
D	Acute cystitis		
E	Malaria		
F	Carcinoma of the kidney		
G	Bladder carcinoma		
H	Bilharzia		
I	Prostate carcinoma		

For each of the cases below, choose the SINGLE most likely cause from the above list of options. Each option may be used once, more than once, or not at all.

1. An 18-year-old female started on oral contraceptives complains of colicky abdominal pain, vomiting and fever. Her urine is positive for red blood cells and protein. She develops progressive weakness in her extremities.

2. A 60-year-old man presents with intermittent colicky loin pain and night sweats. He has profuse haematuria with passage of blood clots. He is noted to have a varicocoele and peripheral oedema. He admits to loss of energy and weight loss.

3. A 25-year-old woman presents with fever and tachycardia. On examination the renal angle is very tender. Her urine is cloudy and blood-stained.

4. A 40-year-old man complains of severe colicky loin pain that radiates to his scrotum. He is noted to have microscopic haematuria. No masses are palpated.

5. A 60-year-old man complains of increased frequency of micturition with suprapubic ache. The urine is cloudy and mahogany brown in colour.

Question 58
Theme: Causes of varicose veins

Options:

A	Pregnancy	J	Retroperitoneal fibrosis
B	Ovarian cyst	K	Deep vein thrombosis
C	Fibroids		
D	Arteriovenous fistula		
E	Intra-abdominal malignancy		
F	Iliac vein thrombosis		
G	Ascites		
H	Klippel-Trenaunay syndrome		
I	Abdominal lymphadenopathy		

For each patient below, choose the SINGLE most likely cause from the above list of options. Each option may be used once, more than once, or not at all.

1. A 60-year-old man complains of pain and swelling in the whole of his right leg. Forced plantar flexion of the leg increases the pain. He is noted to have hard muscles of the leg and lipo-dermatosclerosis.

2. A 30-year-old woman on oral contraceptives presents with dilated tortuous veins crossing her abdomen to join the tributaries of the superior vena cava.

3. A 40-year-old man presents with varicose veins in the lower extremity. He recently underwent orchidectomy for seminoma.

4. A 10-year-old boy presents with tortuous, dilated veins on the lateral side of his left leg. The left leg is slightly longer than the right leg.

5. A 55-year-old man complains of a dull ache in the calves, relieved by lying down. He presents with tortuous, dilated veins on the medial aspect of his lower extremities. He is noted to have splenomegaly, clubbing of his fingers, and small testes.

Question 59
Theme: Causes of haematemesis

Options:

A	Chronic peptic ulceration	J	Angiodysplasia
B	Gastritis	K	Peutz–Jegher syndrome
C	Oesophageal varices	L	Ehlers-Danlos syndrome
D	Mallory–Weiss syndrome		
E	Carcinoma of the oesophagus		
F	Carcinoma of the stomach		
G	Oesophagitis		
H	Haemophilia		
I	Epistaxis		

For each cases below, choose the SINGLE most likely cause from the above list of options. Each option may be used once, more than once, or not at all.

1. A 40-year-old obese man presents with projectile haematemesis after ingestion of a five-course meal and wine.

2. A 50-year-old man presents with massive haematemesis. He is noted to have freckles on his lower lips.

3. A 60-year-old alcoholic man presents with massive haematemesis and shock. He is noted to have finger clubbing and ascites.

4. A 70-year-old man with chronic hoarseness presents with retrosternal chest pain and haematemesis. He has a history of achalasia and has lost 1 stone in weight.

5. A 65-year-old man presents with haematemesis. He is noted to have an enlarged left supraclavicular node, ascites, and anaemia.

Question 60
Theme: Diagnosis of skin lesions

Options:

A	Seborrhoeic keratosis	J	Bowen's disease
B	Malignant melanoma	K	Marjolin's ulcer
C	Café au lait patch		
D	Haemangioma		
E	Campbell de Morgan spot		
F	Keratoacanthoma		
G	Solar keratosis		
H	Basal cell carcinoma		
I	Squamous cell carcinoma		

For each presentation below, choose the SINGLE most likely diagnosis from the above list of options. Each option may be used once, more than once, or not at all.

1. A 60-year-old man presents with a persistent itchy ulcer on his right cheek. He has had this ulcer for years. The edges are rolled with a central scab that falls off and reforms. The local lymph nodes are not enlarged.

2. A 65-year-old farmer presents with a grey thickened patch of skin on the rim of his left ear. The 1 cm lesion is painless, raised, firm, and has not changed in size over many years.

3. A 40-year-old woman presents with a rapidly growing 1 cm lump in the skin of her wrist. The lump is the same colour as her skin but the centre is necrotic. It is freely mobile and rubbery in consistency with a hard core.

4. A newborn baby presents with several, 2 cm, pale brown macules on the back.

5. A 20-year-old man presents with a chronic paronychia. On examination, there is an expanding brown pigmentation present beneath the toe-nail with enlargement of local lymph nodes.

Question 61
Theme: Diagnosis of skin infections

Options:

A   Infected sebaceous cyst   J   Scrofula
B   Furunculosis
C   Cellulitis
D   Herpes zoster
E   Carbuncle
F   Erysipelas
G   Hidradenitis suppurativa
H   Infected sinus
I   Skin necrosis

For each case below, choose the SINGLE most likely diagnosis from the above list of options. Each option may be used once, more than once, or not at all.

1. A 55-year-old non-insulin-dependent diabetic man presents with chronic recurrent tender swellings in his groin. These red swellings eventually discharge pus.

2. A 45-year-old gardener presents with fever and swelling over his left cheek. The left side of his face is red, hot, and tender with a raised border.

3. A 60-year-old obese insulin dependent diabetic woman presents with red papules and vesicles along the left preauricular region and mandible. It was preceded by fever.

4. A 70-year-old man with peripheral vascular disease presents with a pinprick-sized hole in the centre of his groin wound following aorto-bifemoral graft. The discharge is serous.

5. A 50-year-old woman presents with a tender 1.5 cm swelling in the preauricular region. There is a punctum seen in the centre. The swelling is tense and smooth and attached to the skin.

Question 62
Theme: The treatment of hearing loss

Options:

A ENT referral for potential mastoidectomy

B ENT referral for potential stapedectomy

C ENT referral for potential grommet insertion

D Bone anchored hearing aid

E Aural toilet

F Betahistidine

G Insertion of Pope wick and sofradex otic drops

H Amoxicillin suspension

I ENT referral for potential tympanoplasty

J Syringing of the ears

K In-the-ear hearing aids

For each patient below, choose the SINGLE most appropriate treatment from the above list of options. Each option may be used once, more than once, or not at all.

1. A 4-year-old boy presents with a 4-month history of persistent conductive hearing loss in both ears. On examination, he has a bulging, amber-yellow tympanic membrane. He denies pain.

2. A 40-year-old woman presents with persistent, unilateral conductive hearing loss following recurrent ear infections. The hearing loss is confirmed to be severe, and on examination the tympanic membrane has a central perforation.

3. A 30-year-old pregnant woman presents with left-sided, conductive hearing loss. She states that she can hear better in a noisy surrounding. On examination, the tympanic membrane is normal.

4. A 70-year-old woman presents with unilateral conductive hearing loss. On examination, there is cerumen in the external auditory meatus.

5. A 5-year-old girl presents with fever, a painful right ear, and deafness. On examination, the tympanic membrane is full and red.

63

Question 63
Theme: Causes of abnormal electrocardiograms

Options:

A Hypokalaemia
B Hyperkalaemia
C Hypocalcaemia
D Hypercalcaemia
E Myocardial ischaemia
F Inferior myocardial infarction
G Acute pulmonary embolism
H Acute pericarditis
I Atrial fibrillation
J Myxoedema
K Digitalis intoxication
L Inferolateral myocardial infarction

For each case below, choose the SINGLE most likely cause of ECG changes from the above list of options. Each option may be used once, more than once, or not at all.

1. A 60-year-old woman taking frusemide is noted to have 'U' waves in leads V3 and V4.

2. A 50-year-old man presents with fever and chest pain. He has a history of angina. His ECG reveals concave elevation of the ST segments in leads II, V5 and V6.

3. A 55-year-old man presents with chest pain and dyspnoea. His ECG reveals 'Q' waves in leads III and AVf and inverted 'T' waves in leads V1–3.

4. A 55-year-old woman who has undergone thyroidectomy is noted to have an ECG with a QT interval of 0.50.

5. A 60-year-old woman presents with hoarseness. She is a smoker and is on prozac. Her pulse rate is 44/min, and her ECG is noted for sinus bradycardia and reduced amplitude of P, QRS and T waves in all leads.

Question 64
Theme: Causes of abdominal masses

Options:

A   Psoas abscess
B   Appendicitis
C   Tuberculosis
D   Crohn's disease
E   Diverticulitis
F   Carcinoma in the sigmoid colon
G   Carcinoma of the caecum
H   Obstruction of the common bile duct by a calculus
I   Carcinoma of the pancreas

J   Ovarian cyst
K   Mesenteric cyst

For each case below, choose the SINGLE most likely cause from the above list of options. Each option may be used once, more than once, or not at all.

1. A 40-year-old man presents with fever, painless jaundice, and a palpable gallbladder.

2. A 30-year-old woman presents with colicky abdominal pain and distension. On examination, a smooth, mobile, spherical mass is palpated in the centre of her abdomen. A fluid thrill is elicited, and the mass is dull to percussion.

3. A 20-year-old man presents with fever, abdominal and back pain and a mass in the right iliac fossa. The swelling is soft, tender, dull, and compressible. It extends below the groin. He denies nausea, vomiting, or diarrhoea.

4. A 50-year-old man presents with a dull ache in the right iliac fossa and diarrhoea. A freely mobile mass is palpated in the right iliac fossa. The rectum is normal, and the faeces contains blood.

5. A 55-year-old man presents with severe, left iliac fossa pain, nausea, and chronic constipation. A tender, sausage-shaped mass is palpated in the left iliac fossa.

Question 65
Theme: Investigation of failure to thrive

Options:

A	Full blood count (FBC)	J	Fasting blood glucose
B	Sweat test	K	Abdominal ultrasound
C	Urinanalysis		
D	Serum electrolytes		
E	Bone films		
F	Thyroid function tests		
G	Buccal smear (females)		
H	Stool culture		
I	Echocardiogram		

For each presentation below, choose the SINGLE most discriminating investigation from the above list of options. Each option may be used once, more than once, or not at all.

1. A small 6-year-old boy on regular salbutamol inhaler presents with nasal obstruction and persistent cough. On examination, he is found to have nasal polyps.

2. A 2-year-old boy presents with anorexia, impaired growth, abdominal distension, abnormal stools, and hypotonia. He is irritable when examined.

3. A 14-year-old girl presents with anorexia. She reports that her appetite is good but cannot seem to gain weight. Her parents describe her as hyperactive and emotional. Her blood pressure is noted to be 130/80, and her pulse rate 108/min.

4. A 5-year-old boy presents with weight loss and nocturnal enuresis. His parents describe him as having profound mood swings. They have attempted to limit his fluid intake at night.

5. A 6-week-old baby presents with failure to thrive. The mother reports, that he takes one hour for feeding with frequent rests. On examination, he is noted to be tachycardic, tachypneic, and have an enlarged liver.

Question 66
Theme: Investigation of loss of consciousness in a child

Options:

A	Full blood count (FBC)	J	Thyroid function tests
B	Serum electrolytes	K	Chest X-ray
C	Serum glucose	L	Blood cultures
D	Urinanalysis		
E	Serum hepatic enzymes and ammonia level		
F	Computed tomography of the head		
G	Toxicology screens		
H	Lumbar puncture		
I	Serum calcium		

For each presentation below, choose the SINGLE most discriminating investigation from the above list of options. Each option may be used once, more than once, or not at all.

1. A 10-month-old baby is brought into casualty after a fall. He is irritable and drowsy. On examination, he is noted to have bruising behind the ears and blood in the ear canal. His blood pressure is labile.

2. A 10-year-old boy presents with delirium, and emesis following an upper respiratory tract infection. He had been treated with paracetamol and aspirin. On examination, he is apyrexial. His bowel habits are normal.

3. A 10-year-old boy is brought into casualty somnolent. On examination, he is noted to have dry mucous membranes and is noted to be breathing in a deep, sighing manner. The mother explains that he had been complaining of abdominal pain.

4. A 14-year-old girl presents to Casualty in a coma. On examination, papilloedema is noted. Her parents report that she had been complaining of headaches.

5. A 10-month-old baby girl presents with pallor, hypotonia, and listlessness. On examination, she is noted to have a full anterior fontanelle.

Question 67
Theme: The treatment of psychiatric disorders

Options:

A Long-term psychotherapy
B Lithium
C Donepezil, a reverse inhibitor of acetylcholinesterase
D Levodopa in combination with a dopa-decarboxylase inhibitor
E Diazepam
F Haloperidol
G Tetrabenazine
H Propranolol
I Disulfiram
J Methadone
K Prozac

For each case below, choose the SINGLE most appropriate treatment from the above list of options. Each option may be used once, more than once, or not at all.

1. A 70-year-old man presents with progressive forgetfulness and mood changes. He has a shuffling gait. The head CT scan shows cortical atrophy and enlarged ventricles.

2. A 60-year-old man presents with a disturbance of voluntary motor function. His face is expressionless. On examination, he has cogwheel rigidity and bradykinesia.

3. A 10-year-old boy presents with brief, repetitive motor tics and is brought in by his parents for shouting obscenities at school.

4. A 40-year-old man presents with ataxia. His wife states that it runs in her husband's family. He is difficult to live with, very irritable, clumsy, and suffers from jerky movements of the legs.

5. A 20-year-old man presents with sweating, muscle twitching, and abdominal cramps. On examination, he has dilated pupils.

Question 68
Theme: Diagnosis of anorectal diseases

Options:

A	Fistulo-in-ano	J	Proctalgia fugax
B	Anorectal abscess	K	Prolapsed rectum
C	Pilonidal sinus	L	Intussusception
D	Perianal haematoma		
E	Perianal warts		
F	Fissure-in-ano		
G	Carcinoma of the rectum		
H	Haemorrhoids		
I	Diverticular disease		

For each patient below, choose the SINGLE most likely diagnosis from the above list of options. Each option may be used once, more than once, or not at all.

1. A 90-year-old female presents with a large lump in her anus. It appeared after defecation. The lump is red with concentric folds of mucosa around a central pit and is nontender.

2. A 50-year-old woman presents to her GP with severe rectal pain. It is worse at night and lasts minutes to hours. The rectal examination is normal.

3. A 39-year-old Italian man presents to his GP with a painful bottom. On examination, the gluteal cleft over the midline of the sacrum, and coccyx is red and tender.

4. A 30-year-old man presents with anal pain, discharge and itching. On examination there are multiple openings 2 cm behind and to the right of the anus.

5. A 29-year-old mother of two presents with pain on defecation with blood staining of the toilet paper. On examination, she has a split in the skin posterior to the anus and a small skin tag at the lower end.

Question 69
Theme: Diagnosis of rectal bleeding

Options:

A	Carcinoma of the colon	J	Fistulae in Crohn's disease
B	Proctitis		
C	Carcinoma of the rectum		
D	Haemorrhoids		
E	Ulcerative colitis		
F	Diverticular disease		
G	Peptic ulceration		
H	Fissure-in-ano		
I	Carcinoma of the anus		

For each patient below, choose the SINGLE most likely diagnosis from the above list of options. Each option may be used once, more than once, or not at all.

1. A 30-year-old man presents with painless rectal bleeding mixed with mucus. He has a history of intermittent diarrhoea. On examination, there is no evidence of perianal disease.

2. A 40-year-old man presents with painless melena. On examination, the anus and rectum are normal. He denies weight loss. He drinks and smokes heavily.

3. A 25-year-old man presents with anal pain, bloody discharge, and mucus. On examination, there are multiple puckered scars around the anus.

4. A 50-year-old man passes 500 ml of fresh blood from his rectum. He describes a need to defecate but instead of passing stool, he passed blood. He has chronic, left-sided abdominal discomfort. He denies weight loss and has no palpable masses.

5. A 70-year-old man presents with painless rectal bleeding. The blood is streaked on his stool. He complains of tenesmus. A soft, fixed mass is palpated on digital rectal exam. There are no palpable inguinal lymph nodes.

Question 70
Theme: The treatment of medical emergencies

Options:

A	Cardioversion	J	Intramuscular adrenaline
B	Cricothyroidotomy	K	Intravenous amino-
C	Needle thoracocentesis		phylline
D	Needle pericardiocentesis		
E	Insertion of chest drain		
F	Endotracheal intubation		
G	Defibrillation		
H	Needle aspiration		
I	Intravenous heparin		

For each case below, choose the SINGLE most appropriate treatment from the above list of options. Each option may be used once, more than once, or not at all.

1. A 45-year-old woman presents with acute dyspnoea and stridor. Her tongue is swollen.

2. A 20-year-old student presents with respiratory distress and pleuritic pain. On examination, he has distended neck veins and no breath sounds over the right lung field.

3. A 30-year-old man presents with chest pain. He has distended neck veins and muffled heart sounds. His blood pressure is 80/50.

4. A 55-year-old woman presents with stridor and difficulty swallowing following thyroidectomy. On examination, she has a tense swelling over the surgical site.

5. A 30-year-old female presents with acute dyspnoea and pleuritic pain. Her regular medications include salbutamol inhaler and an oral contraceptive. Her respiratory rate is 30, with a small volume rapid pulse rate of 110 and a blood pressure of 80/50. She has a raised jugular venous pressure. The chest X-ray is normal. Her electrocardiogram shows sinus tachycardia.

Question 71
Theme: Diagnosis of medical syndromes

Options:

A   Pendred's syndrome
B   Patterson-Brown Kelly syndrome
C   Plummer-Vinson syndrome
D   Reiter's syndrome
E   Waterhouse-Friedrichsen syndrome
F   Shieie's syndrome
G   Peutz–Jegher syndrome
H   Fanconi's syndrome
I   Zollinger–Ellison syndrome

J   Reye's syndrome
K   Mallory–Weiss syndrome
L   Sjögren's syndrome
M   Felty's syndrome

For each patient below, choose the SINGLE most likely diagnosis from the above list of options. Each option may be used once, more than once, or not at all.

1. A 50-year-old man presents with a low white count and anaemia. He is noted to have splenomegaly. He takes diclofenac for his arthritis.

2. A 55-year-old man is noted to have freckles on his lips and occasional rectal bleeding.

3. A 20-year-old man presents with bone pain, polyuria, and polydipsia. He is noted to have glycosuria and aminoaciduria.

4. A 25-year-old man presents with arthritis, urethritis, conjunctivitis, and keratoderma blenorrhagicum.

5. A 50-year-old woman with rheumatoid arthritis complains of diminished lacrimation and salivation.

Question 72
Theme: Causes of potential drug toxicity through drug interaction

Options:

A	Loop diuretics	J	Verapamil
B	Allopurinol	K	Amiodarone
C	NSAIDs	L	Chloramphenicol
D	Alcohol	M	Omeprazole
E	Erythromycin		
F	Aminophylline		
G	Thiazide diuretics		
H	Ranitidine		
I	Cimetidine		

For each case below, choose the SINGLE most likely cause from the above list of options. Each option may be used once, more than once, or not at all.

1. A 40-year-old manic depressive is noted to have high serum levels of lithium and profound hypokalaemia. His GP had started him on an antihypertensive.

2. A 55-year-old man on warfarin presents with epistaxis. His INR is noted to be 5. His other medications include glipizide, tagamet, and paracetamol.

3. A 40-year-old woman on carbamazepine for trigeminal neuralgia now presents with severe dizziness. She was recently started on an antibiotic course.

4. A 50-year-old man taking phenytoin for epilepsy now presents with ataxia, slurred speech, and blurred vision. His medications include carbamazepine, tagamet, and allopurinol.

5. A 55-year-old diabetic on metformin presents with lactic acidosis. His medications include erythromycin and paracetamol. He also drinks heavily.

Question 73
Theme: Diagnosis of abnormal childhood development

Options:

A Klinefelter's syndrome
B Turner's syndrome
C Testicular feminisation syndrome
D Marfan's syndrome
E Adrenogenital syndrome
F Homocystinuria
G Achondroplasia
H Down's syndrome
I Duchenne muscular dystrophy
J Spina bifida
K Cerebral palsy
L Osteogenesis imperfecta
M Acromegaly

For each case below, choose the SINGLE most likely diagnosis from the above list of options. Each option may be used once, more than once, or not at all.

1. An 18-month-old boy presents to the GP for late walking and difficulty climbing stairs. On examination, the boy has a lumbar lordosis and calf hypertrophy.

2. A 14-year-old girl presents to the GP for absence of periods. On exam she is petite with no breast development. Other noted features include pterygium colli and cubitus valgus.

3. A 15-year-old boy presents to his GP with a sore throat. He is tall for his age and is noted to have long limbs and small testicles.

4. A 16-year-old girl presents to her GP with flat feet. She is tall for her age and is noted to have a high arched palate and a long arm span.

5. A 6-year-old boy presents to his GP with short stature. He has a large skull, a prominent forehead, and a saddle-shaped nose. The back is lordotic.

Question 74
Theme: Diagnosis of normal developmental milestones

Options:

A   3 months
B   6 months
C   9 months
D   12 months
E   18 months
F   2 years
G   3 years
H   4 years
I   5 years

J   6 years
K   7 years

For each case below, choose the SINGLE most appropriate age from the above list of options. Each option may be used once, more than once, or not at all.

1. A child is asked to copy figures. She can successfully draw a square and triangle but has difficulty with copying a diamond.

2. A mother is concerned that her baby is not walking yet. He is sitting unsupported and is babbling contentedly. He holds a pencil in a scissor grasp and transfers the pencil between his hands prior to placing it in his mouth.

3. A child is asked to copy figures. She can only copy a circle. She can climb up stairs one foot per step and builds a tower of 9 cubes.

4. A child is asked to copy figures. She can copy a circle and a cross. She can stand on one foot for 5 seconds and climbs up and down stairs one foot per step.

5. A mother is concerned that her baby is not talking yet. He walks around furniture and can stand alone for a few seconds. He holds objects in a pincer grasp.

Question 75
Theme: Diagnosis of childhood seizures

Options:

A   Grand mal
B   Infantile spasm
C   Febrile convulsions
D   Status epilepticus
E   Petit mal
F   Temporal lobe seizure
G   Jacksonian seizure
H   Tuberous sclerosis
I   Neurofibromatosis

J   Sturge-Weber syndrome
K   Benign paroxysmal vertigo

For each case below, choose the SINGLE most likely diagnosis from the above list of options. Each option may be used once, more than once, or not at all.

1. A 9-year-old boy is brought to the GP for daydreaming at school. The attack is reproduced by encouraging the child to hyperventilate. The child becomes inattentive for 5 seconds, and the eyes roll up.

2. A 10-year-old boy presents to the GP with worsening seizures. The attacks begin with a cry and continuous muscle spasm, followed by jerking and tongue-biting. The child then drifts into unconsciousness.

3. A 3-year-old girl presents to the GP with ear-ache and seizures. She is pyrexial and on examination, has acute otitis media. The seizure is described as lasting for 5 minutes with jerky movements of the limbs.

4. A 12-year-old boy presents to his GP with convulsions that are described to start in his thumb and progress along the same side of his body.

5. An 8-year-old boy presents with a history of epilepsy and mental retardation. He is noted to have a butterfly distribution of warty lesions over his nose and cheeks.

Question 76
Theme: Investigation of childhood endocrine and metabolic disorders

Options:

A   Full blood count (FBC)
B   Serum electrolytes
C   Serum ADH levels
D   Serum growth hormone levels
E   Detection of phenylketones in the urine
F   Thyroid function tests
G   Detection of galactose in the urine
H   Serum ACTH levels
I   High serum blood glucose
J   Low serum blood glucose
K   Detection of cystine in the urine
L   Plasma cortisol levels

For each case below, choose the SINGLE most discriminating investigation from the above list of options. Each option may be used once, more than once, or not at all.

1. A 1-month-old baby presents with poor feeding and lethargy. On examination he has an umbilical hernia and an enlarged tongue.

2. A newborn female is noted to have an enlarged clitoris and fused labia.

3. A 13-year-old obese girl with a history of asthma and eczema presents with amenorrhoea. Her blood pressure is noted to be 130/80.

4. A 1-month-old baby presents with vomiting, jaundice, and hepatomegaly. The baby is worse after feeding.

5. An 8-year-old boy presents to the GP with short stature. He complains of constant thirst and is noted to pass huge volumes of colourless urine.

Question 77
Theme: Investigation of liver disease

Options:

A   Mitochondrial antibodies
B   Serum iron and total iron-
    binding capacity
C   Serum copper and
    caeruloplasmin
D   Serum bilirubin and liver
    function tests
E   HBs antigen
F   Antibodies to HCV
G   Antibodies against nuclei and
    actin
H   Antibodies to HAV
I   Gamma-glutamyl transferase
    level

J   Alpha-1-antitrypsin

For each presentation below, choose the SINGLE most discriminating investigation from the above list of options. Each option may be used once, more than once, or not at all.

1. A 60-year-old man with emphysema presents with liver disease. His sputum is purulent and found to contain elastases and proteases.

2. A 50-year-old woman presents with pruritus and jaundice. She complains of dry eyes and mouth. On examination she has xanthelasma and hepatosplenomegaly.

3. A 50-year-old well-bronzed man presents with a loss of libido. He is noted to have hepatomegaly. He takes humulin and actrapid insulin.

4. A 22-year-old man presents with tremor and dysarthria. On examination, he is noted to have a greenish-brown pigment at the corneoscleral junction.

5. A 30-year-old woman presents with acute hepatitis. She is pyrexial, jaundiced, with hepatosplenomegaly, bruising, and migratory polyarthritis. She is noted to have a goitre.

Question 78
Theme: Causes of back pain

Options:

A	Multiple myeloma	J	Spinal stenosis
B	Secondary prostate disease	K	Paget's disease
C	Osteomyelitis	L	Osteoarthritis
D	Ankylosing spondylitis		
E	Sarcoidosis		
F	Lupus		
G	Reiter's disease		
H	Lumbar prolapse and sciatica		
I	Spondylolisthesis		

For each presentation below, choose the SINGLE most likely cause from the above list of options. Each option may be used once, more than once, or not at all.

1. A 30-year-old female complains of sudden and severe back pain. Her back has 'gone'. She walks with a compensated scoliosis. On examination, she has pain from the buttock to her ankle and sensory loss over the sole of her left foot and calf.

2. A 50-year-old man presents with back pain radiating down both his legs. The pain is aggravated by walking and relieved by resting or leaning forward. On exam he has limited straight-leg raise and absent ankle reflexes.

3. A 50-year-old woman presents with backache. She is noted to have a normocytic, normochromic anaemia and a high erythrocyte sedimentation rate.

4. A 60-year-old man presents with lumbar spine bone pain and pain in his hips. He is noted to have an elevated serum alkaline phosphatase of 1000 IU/L. The calcium and phosphate levels are normal. He is hard of hearing.

5. A 20-year-old man complains of lower back pain radiating down the back of both his legs. On X-ray, the vertebrae are square and tramline. His ESR is elevated.

Question 79
Theme: Investigation of urinary tract obstruction

Options:

A   Excretion urography
B   Ultrasonography
C   Dynamic scintigraphy
D   Cystourethroscopy
E   Plain KUB film
F   Pressure-flow studies
G   Retrograde ureterography
H   Urethrography
I   Serum urea and electrolytes

J   Urinanalysis
K   Mid-stream specimen for culture

For each presentation below, choose the SINGLE most discriminating investigation from the above list of options. Each option may be used, once, more than once, or not at all.

1. A 65-year-old diabetic man presents with a painless distended bladder. On digital rectal exam, his prostate is not enlarged.

2. A 40-year-old man presents with severe, colicky loin pain radiating to his testicle. Plain abdominal X-ray is unremarkable. He has microscopic haematuria.

3. A 50-year-old man presents with severe oliguria, post kidney transplant.

4. A 60-year-old man post-thyroidectomy presents with painful urinary retention. There is some difficulty in catheterisation, with a 900 ml residual. Digital rectal exam reveals a smooth, enlarged prostate.

5. A 60-year-old man presents with malaise, back pain, normochromic anaemia, uraemia, and a high ESR. He has known carcinoma of the colon.

Question 80
Theme: Diagnosis of renal failure

Options:

A	Goodpasture's syndrome	J	Drugs causing nephrotic syndrome
B	Amyloidosis		
C	Systemic lupus erythematosus	K	Haemolytic uraemic syndrome
D	Polyarteritis nodosa		
E	Wegener's granulomatosis	L	Acute tubulo-interstitial nephritis
F	Systemic sclerosis		
G	Post-streptoccocal glomerulonephritis		
H	Multiple myeloma		
I	Diabetic glomerulosclerosis		

For each case below, choose the SINGLE most likely diagnosis from the above list of options. Each option may be used once, more than once, or not at all.

1. A 4-year-old boy presents to the GP with bloody diarrhoea and haematuria. His full blood count reveals a leukocytosis, haemolytic anaemia, and thrombocytopaenia.

2. A 50-year-old woman presents with fever, polyarthralgia, a skin rash and oliguria. She is a diabetic and suffers from arthritis. She takes insulin and allopurinol.

3. A 50-year-old man with a history of heart failure now presents in renal failure. On examination, he has an enlarged tongue, hepatosplenomegaly, and peripheral oedema. He has heavy urinary protein loss and low serum albumin.

4. A 55-year-old man presents in acute renal failure. He suffers from rhinitis. Round lung shadows are noted on chest X-ray.

5. A 20-year-old man presents with rapidly progressive renal failure. He describes a recent history of cough, fatigue, and occasional haemoptysis. His chest X-ray reveals blotchy shadows.

Question 81
Theme: The treatment of renal disease

Options:

A	Cyclophosphamide	I	Albumin infusion with mannitol
B	Bendrofluazide		
C	Haemodialysis	J	Salt restriction with frusemide
D	Renal transplantation		
E	Immunosuppressive treatment and plasmapharesis	K	Peritoneal dialysis
		L	Corticosteroids
F	Fluid and protein restriction		
G	Continuous arteriovenous haemofiltration		
H	Withdrawal of offending drug		

For each case below, choose the SINGLE most appropriate treatment from the above list of options. Each option may be used once, more than once, or not at all.

1. A 20-year-old man presents with dyspnoea, haemoptysis, and acute renal failure. He has serum anti-glomerular basement membrane antibodies.

2. A 55-year-old man is noted to have a nasal septal perforation, hypertension and glomerulonephritis. The chest X-ray reveals multiple nodules.

3. A 60-year-old man presents with fits, confusion, pulmonary oedema and anuria. His serum urea is 50 mmol/L, and his potassium is 8 mmol/L. He has a history of MI and previous bowel resection.

4. A 5-year-old boy presents with generalised oedema. On examination, he is noted to have facial oedema, ascites, and scrotal oedema. His urine is frothy with the presence of proteins and hyaline casts. His serum albumin is 24 g/L, and the serum cholesterol is raised.

5. A 7-year-old boy presents with bright red urine and oedema of the eyelids. His blood pressure is noted to be high. The urine reveals white cells, red cells, granular casts, and protein.

Question 82
Theme: Diagnosis of childhood malignancy

Options:

A	Wilm's tumour	J	Astrocytoma
B	Neuroblastoma	K	Medulloblastoma
C	Acute lymphoblastic leukaemia	L	Brain stem glioma
D	Acute myeloid leukaemia		
E	Rhabdomyosarcoma		
F	Ewing's sarcoma		
G	Osteosarcoma		
H	Hodgkin's disease		
I	Non-Hodgkin's lymphoma		

For each patient below, choose the SINGLE most likely diagnosis from the above list of options. Each option may be used once, more than once, or not at all.

1. A 4-year-old boy presents to the GP with a unilateral abdominal mass noted while bathing. He has microscopic haematuria. Intravenous urogram shows a distorted kidney.

2. A 3-year-old boy presents to the GP with a unilateral abdominal mass and bone pain. He is irritable. The abdominal X-ray shows calcifications within the mass.

3. A 13-year-old girl presents with a painless neck lump. Chest X-ray reveals hilar adenopathy. Fine needle aspirate of the neck lump reveals Reed-Sternberg cells.

4. A 14-year-old boy presents with a painless neck lump and a painful abdominal mass. Investigations reveal a normochromic, normocytic anaemia and a raised ESR. Fine needle aspirate of the neck lump reveals centroblastic B-cells.

5. A 5-year-old boy presents with headache and vomiting. On fundoscopic examination, he is noted to have papilloedema. CT scan reveals a mass arising from the roof of the fourth ventricle causing obstructive hydrocephalus.

Question 83
Theme: Diagnosis of chronic joint pain

Options:

A	Gout	I	Still's disease
B	Septic arthritis	J	Multiple myeloma
C	Rheumatoid arthritis	K	Sjögren's syndrome
D	Osteoarthritis		
E	Pyrophosphate arthropathy		
F	Systemic lupus erythematosus		
G	Systemic sclerosis		
H	Polymyositis		

For each case below, choose the SINGLE most likely diagnosis from the above list of options. Each option may be used once, more than once, or not at all.

1. A 70-year-old woman complains of arthritis in the fingers and big toe. On examination, she has bony swellings of the first carpometacarpal joints, at the proximal interphalangeal joints and has an affected metatarsophalangeal joint.

2. A 45-year-old woman presents with swellings and stiffness of her fingers. On examination, she has sausage-like fingers with flexion deformities. She is noted to have a beaked nose. She takes losec. X-ray of her hands reveal deposits of calcium around the fingers and erosion of the tufts of the distal phalanges.

3. A 40-year-old woman complains of arthritic hands, weakness in her arms and difficulty swallowing. She has trouble carrying her shopping. On examination, the small joints of her hands are swollen. Blood tests reveal a raised ESR and a normocytic anaemia. Serum antinuclear antibodies and rheumatoid factor tests are positive.

4. A 50-year-old woman on throxine for hypothroidism presents with stiff swollen knees. Aspiration of the synovial fluid reveals positively birefringent crystals.

5. An elderly man presents with a red, warm, swollen metatarsal phalangeal joint following a right total hip replacement operation.

Question 84
Theme: Causes of finger clubbing

Options:

A Bronchial carcinoma	J Inflammatory bowel disease
B Bronchiectasis	
C Lung abscess	K Coeliac disease
D Empyema	L GI lymphoma
E Cryptogenic fibrosing alveolitis	
F Mesothelioma	
G Cyanotic heart disease	
H Subacute bacterial endocarditis	
I Cirrhosis	

For each presentation below, choose the SINGLE most likely associative cause from the above list of options. Each option may be used once, more than once, or not at all.

1. A 35-year-old heroin addict presents with fever, night sweats and haematuria. On exam he is noted to have a heart murmur and finger clubbing.

2. A 50-year-old farmer is noted to have a dry cough, exertional dyspnoea, weight loss, arthalgia, and finger clubbing. On X-ray, there are bilateral diffuse reticulonodular shadowing at the bases.

3. A 60-year-old man presents with severe chest pain, dyspnoea, and finger clubbing. He admits to asbestos exposure 20 years ago. He denies smoking. The chest X-ray reveals a unilateral pleural effusion.

4. A 30-year-old woman presents with fever, diarrhoea, and crampy abdominal pain. She is noted to have finger clubbing, anal fissures, and a skin tag.

5. A 50-year-old man presents with haematemesis. He is noted to have finger clubbing, gynaecomastia, and spider naevi.

Question 85
Theme: Causes of headache

Options:

A	Meningitis	J	Otitis media
B	Migraine headache	K	Transient ischaemic attack
C	Cluster headache		
D	Tension headache		
E	Subarachnoid haemorrhage		
F	Sinusitis		
G	Benign intracranial hypertension		
H	Cervical spondylosis		
I	Giant-cell arteritis		

For each case below, choose the SINGLE most likely cause from the above list of options. Each option may be used once, more than once, or not at all.

1. A 25-year-old female presents with episodes of unilateral throbbing headache, nausea, and vomiting. She states that it is aggravated by light. The episodes seem to occur prior to her menstruation.

2. A 40-year-old man presents with severe pain around his right eye, with eyelid swelling lasting 20 minutes. He has had several attacks during the past weeks. The attacks are worse at night.

3. A 10-year-old boy presents with fever, headache, left eye pain, and swelling. He described his vision as blurry. He has recently recovered from a cold.

4. A 60-year-old female presents with bitemporal headache, unilateral blurry vision, and pain on combing her hair. Her ESR is elevated.

5. A 30-year-old obese female presents with headache and diplopia. On examination, she has papilloedema. She is alert with no focal symptoms and signs.

Question 86
Theme: Causes of facial nerve palsy

Options:

A	Bell's palsy	J	Cerebrovascular accident
B	Parotid tumour		
C	Ramsay Hunt syndrome	K	Longitudinal temporal bone fracture
D	Multiple sclerosis		
E	Facial nerve schwannoma	L	Malignant otitis externa
F	Sarcoid		
G	Transverse temporal bone fracture		
H	Suppurative otitis media		
I	Guillain–Barré syndrome		

For each case below, choose the SINGLE most likely cause from the above list of options. Each option may be used once, more than once, or not at all.

1. A 40-year-old man presents with facial pain, a droop to the side of his face, and a preauricular facial swelling.

2. A 30-year-old man who has sustained a blow to the back of his head presents with facial nerve palsy and haemotympanum.

3. A 55-year-old woman presents with a right-sided lower motor neuron facial nerve palsy and sensorineural hearing loss. She is noted to have vesicles in her right ear.

4. A 50-year-old diabetic man presents with a unilateral facial nerve palsy and severe earache. On examination, he has granulation tissue deep in the external auditory meatus.

5. A 40-year-old woman presents with unilateral optic neuritis and a facial nerve palsy.

Question 87
Theme: Diagnosis of liver disease

Options:

A Budd–Chiari syndrome
B Cholestasis
C Haemolytic jaundice
D Hepatocellular failure
E Acute hepatitis C
F Acute hepatitis B
G Acute hepatitis A
H Primary biliary cirrhosis
I Alcoholic hepatitis

J Haemochromatosis
K Wilson's disease
L Hepatocellular carcinoma

For each patient below, choose the SINGLE most likely diagnosis from the above list of options. Each option may be used once, more than once, or not at all.

1. A 22-year-old woman presents with right upper quadrant abdominal pain and ascites. On examination, she has hepatomegaly. Diagnostic liver scintiscan shows maximum uptake in the caudate lobe alone. Her regular medications include the oral contraceptive pill and prozac.

2. A 50-year-old woman presents with hepatomegaly and darkened skin pigmentation. She admits to drinking heavily. She is noted to have glycosuria.

3. A 40-year-old man presents with jaundice. He was started on chlorpromazine for intractable hiccups three weeks ago.

4. A 50-year-old man presents with tender hepatomegaly and fever. His blood tests reveal an elevated MCV and an elevated gamma-glutamyl transpeptidase.

5. A 40-year-old woman presents with tender hepatomegaly and weight loss. She takes the oral contraceptive and atenolol. She is noted to have a raised alpha-fetoprotein.

Question 88
Theme: Diagnosis of cardiovascular disease

Options:

A	Aortic regurgitation	J	Fallot's tetralogy
B	Mitral stenosis	K	Patent ductus arteriosus
C	Mitral regurgitation	L	Coarctation of the aorta
D	Aortic stenosis	M	Eisenmenger's syndrome
E	Atrial myxoma		
F	Tricuspid regurgitation		
G	Pulmonary stenosis		
H	Atrial septal defect		
I	Ventricular septal defect		

For each pateint below, choose the SINGLE most likely diagnosis from the above list of options. Each option may be used once, more than once, or not at all.

1. A 35-year-old pregnant woman presents to her GP for her first prenatal check-up. He notes that her blood pressure differs in both arms and is lower in the legs.

2. A 13-year-old boy presents with dyspnoea and short stature. He is noted to have finger clubbing. His chest X-ray reveals a boot-shaped heart and a large aorta.

3. A preterm baby presents with tachypnoea and expiratory grunting. The baby is noted to have a continuous machinery-like murmur in the second left intercostal space and posteriorly. The ECG is normal.

4. A 33-year-old woman with Marfan's syndrome is noted to have a fixed wide split of the second heart sound. The ECG shows a partial right bundle branch block with right axis deviation and right ventricular hypertrophy.

5. A 40-year-old drug addict is noted to have a pansystolic murmur at the bottom of the sternum. Giant 'cv' waves are present in the jugular venous pulse.

Question 89
Theme: Diagnosis of peripheral vascular disease

Options:

A	Acute ischaemia of the legs	J	Cardiovascular syphilis
B	Chronic ischaemia of the legs	K	Abdominal aneurysm
C	Intermittent claudication		
D	Raynaud's phenomenon		
E	Ischaemic foot		
F	Dissecting aortic aneurysm		
G	Takayasu's syndrome		
H	Kawasaki disease		
I	Thromboangiitis obliterans		

For each patient below, choose the SINGLE most likely diagnosis from the above list of options. Each option may be used once, more than once, or not at all.

1. A 23-year-old female presents with paresthesias and loss of distal pulses in her arms. She is noted to be hypertensive. She describes feeling unwell a month prior with fever and night sweats.

2. A 20-year-old male smoker is noted to have intense rubor of the feet and absent foot pulses. On examination, he has an amputated right second toe.

3. A 25-year-old female complains of intermittent pain in her fingers. She describes episodes of numbness and burning of the fingers. She wears gloves whenever she leaves the house.

4. A 60-year-old smoker presents with cramp-like pain in the calves relieved by rest and non-healing ulcers. On examination, he has cold extremities with lack of hair around the ankles and absent distal pulses.

5. A 70-year-old man presents with an acutely painful, pale, paralysed and pulseless left leg. He is noted to have atrial fibrillation.

Question 90
Theme: Causes of chest pain

Options:

A	Dissecting aortic aneurysm	I	Mediastinitis
B	Myocardial infarction	J	Enlargening aortic aneurysm
C	Angina pectoris		
D	Pericarditis	K	Tension pneumothorax
E	Pulmonary embolism	L	Pleurisy
F	Costochondritis	M	Dry pleurisy
G	Gastrooesophageal reflux disease		
H	Spontaneous pneumothorax		

For each presentation below, choose the SINGLE most likely cause from the above list of options. Each option may be used once, more than once, or not at all.

1. A 55-year-old man presents with sudden onset of severe and central chest pain radiating to the back. Peripheral pulses are absent. There are no ECG changes. The chest X-ray shows a widened mediastinum.

2. A 20-year-old man recently back from a holiday in the Caribbean presents with left-sided chest discomfort and dyspnoea. On chest X-ray, there is a small area devoid of lung markings in the apex of the left lung.

3. A 50-year-old man recently back from a business trip in Hong Kong presents with sudden onset of breathlessness, haemoptysis, and chest pain. He is brought into Casualty in shock. His chest X-ray is normal. The ECG shows sinus tachycardia.

4. A 40-year-old man presents with central, crushing chest pain that radiates to the jaw. The pain occurred while jogging around the local park. The pain was alleviated with rest. The ECG is normal.

5. A 50-year-old woman with ovarian carcinoma presents with right-sided chest pain. The chest X-ray shows obliteration of the right costophrenic angle.

Question 91
Theme: Causes of delirium

Options:

A	Hepatic failure	J	Brain tumour
B	Renal failure	K	Subarachnoid
C	Hypoxia		haemorrhage
D	Pellagra	L	Drug intoxication
E	Wernicke–Korsakoff syndrome	M	Brain abscess
F	Beriberi		
G	Hypoglycaemia		
H	Alcohol withdrawal		
I	Drug withdrawal		

For each presentation below, choose the SINGLE most likely cause from the above list of options. Each option may be used once, more than once, or not at all.

1. A 60-year-old man presents with confusion, restlessness, and walks with a broad-based gait. On examination, he has nystagmus and bilateral lateral rectus palsies and smells of alcohol.

2. A 40-year-old man taking isoniazid for tuberculosis now presents with dermatitis, diarrhoea, and dementia.

3. A 30-year-old man presents with pinpoint pupils and delirium. He is noted to have a nasal septal perforation.

4. A 35-year-old man presents with fever, delirium and fits. He has a history of chronic sinusitis. On examination, he has asymmetrical pupils and a rising blood pressure. There are no external signs of head trauma.

5. A 55-year-old man presents with seizures and hallucinations. He is tachycardic with a low blood pressure. He insists there are insects crawling over his body. He has a history of alcoholism.

Question 92
Theme: Causes of pneumonia

Options:

A	Chlamydia psittaci	J	Aspergillus fumigatus
B	Streptococcus pneumoniae	K	Cytomegalovirus
C	Mycoplasma pneumoniae	L	Actinomyces israelii
D	Haemophilus influenzae	M	Klebsiella pneumoniae
E	Staphylococcus aureus		
F	Legionella pneumophila		
G	Coxiella burnetti		
H	Pseudomonas aeruginosa		
I	Pneumocystis carinii		

For each case below, choose the SINGLE most likely cause from the above list of options. Each option may be used once, more than once, or not at all.

1. A pet-shop owner presents with high, swinging fever, cough, and malaise. He has scanty rose spots over his abdomen. The chest X-ray reveals diffuse pneumonia.

2. A 70-year-old alcoholic man presents with sudden onset of purulent productive cough. The chest X-ray shows consolidation of the left upper lobe.

3. A 10-year-old boy with cystic fibrosis presents with pneumonia.

4. A 30-year-old man with AIDS presents with fever, dry cough, and dyspnoea. The X-ray shows diffuse, bilateral, alveolar, and interstitial shadowing beginning in the perihilar regions and spreading outward.

5. A 20-year-old male IVDA presents with breathlessness and cough. The X-ray reveals patchy areas of consolidation with abscess formation.

Question 93
Theme: Causes of visual disturbance

Options:

A	*Chlamydia trachomatis*	J	Pituitary neoplasm
B	Side-effect of medication	K	Oculomotor nerve lesion
C	Giant-cell arteritis	L	Abducens nerve lesion
D	Diabetic retinopathy		
E	Multiple sclerosis		
F	Vitamin B$_{12}$ deficiency		
G	Horner's syndrome		
H	Neurosyphilis		
I	Myasthenia gravis		

For each case below, choose the SINGLE most likely cause from the above list of options. Each option may be used once, more than once, or not at all.

1. A 40-year-old woman presents with blurry vision. On examination, when asked to look to her left, the left eye develops nystagmus, and the right eye fails to adduct. When asked to look to her right, the left eye fails to adduct.

2. A 30-year-old woman is noted to have a small, irregular pupil that is fixed to light but constricts on convergence. Her fasting blood glucose is 5 mmol/L.

3. A 24-year-old man presents with unilateral pupillary constriction with slight ptosis and enophthalmos. He is noted to have a cervical rib on X-ray.

4. A 25-year-old man who has sustained head injury in an RTA presents with diplopia on lateral gaze. On examination, he has a convergent squint with diplopia when looking to the left side.

5. A 40-year-old diabetic man presents with a unilateral complete ptosis. The eye is noted to be facing down and out. The pupil is spared.

Question 94
Theme: Causes of depression

Options:

A	Premenstrual syndrome	J	Manic-depressive
B	Puerperal affective disorder		disorder
C	Major depression	K	Drug abuse
D	Drug-induced depression	L	Vitamin and mineral
E	Bereavement reaction		disorders
F	Hypothyroidism		
G	Cushing's syndrome		
H	Hyperparathyroidism		
I	Porphyria		

For each case below, choose the SINGLE most likely cause from the above list of options. Each option may be used once, more than once, or not at all.

1. A 23-year-old female complains of irritability and constant depression. She has thought about suicide. She has trouble sleeping and has lost her appetite.

2. A 20-year-old female complains of episodes of irritability and depression. She also complains of monthly bloating and tension.

3. A 30-year-old female complains of depression, lethargy, constipation, and weight gain. She also suffers from menorrhagia.

4. A 40-year-old woman presents with depression and weight gain. She complains of back pain and excessive thirst. Her menstrual period lasts for 3 days and sometimes she skips a cycle. On examination, she is obese with acne and peripheral oedema.

5. A 30-year-old female on oral contraceptives presents with colicky abdominal pain, vomiting, anxiety, and depression. She is noted to be hypertensive. On standing, the urine turns deep red.

Question 95
Theme: Investigation of dementia

Options:

A Chest X-ray
B Serum calcium level
C TSH levels and serum T4
D Full blood count and film
E Electroencephalogram
F Lumbar puncture
G Serum urea
H Liver function tests
I Computerised tomography (CT scan)

J Serum glucose
K VDRL
L HIV serology
M Serum copper and caeruloplasmin
N Dietary history
O Drug levels

For each case below, choose the SINGLE most discriminating investigation from the above list of options. Each option may be used once, more than once, or not at all.

1. A 50-year-old woman who underwent thyroidectomy a week prior now presents with dementia. She also complains of peri-oral tingling.

2. A 70-year-old man presents with progressive dementia and tremor. On examination, he has extensor plantar reflexes and Argyll Robertson pupils.

3. A 40-year-old man with a history of epilepsy presents with progressive dementia with fluctuating levels of consciousness. On examination, he has unequal pupils.

4. A 30-year-old homosexual man presents with weight loss, chronic diarrhoea and progressive dementia. On examination, he has purple papules on his legs.

5. A 30-year-old man presents with sweating, agitation, tremors, and dementia. He admits to binge drinking.

Question 96
Theme: Causes of shock

Options:

A	Pulmonary embolism	J	Ectopic pregnancy
B	Myocardial ischaemia	K	Addisonian crisis
C	Cardiac tamponade	L	Hypothyroidism
D	Trauma	M	Acute pancreatitis
E	Burns		
F	Sepsis		
G	Anaphylaxis		
H	Major surgery		
I	Ruptured aortic aneurysm		

For each patient below, choose the SINGLE most likely cause from the above list of options. Each option may be used once, more than once, or not at all.

1. A 50-year-old man arrives to Casualty in shock. His BP is 80/50. His heart sounds are muffled. His jugular venous pressure is noted to increase with inspiration.

2. A 30-year-old woman presents to Casualty in respiratory distress and shock. She is noted to have stridor. Her lips are swollen and blue.

3. A 55-year-old man presents to Casualty with severe abdominal pain, vomiting and shock. The pain is in the upper abdomen and radiates to the back. He takes diuretics. The abdomen is rigid, and the X-ray shows absent psoas shadow.

4. A 40-year-old woman presents to Casualty in shock with continuous abdominal pain radiating to her back. The abdomen is rigid with an expansile abdominal mass.

5. A 35-year-old woman presents to Casualty in shock with a BP of 80/50 and tachycardia. She is confused and weak. Her husband states that she forgot to take her prednisolone tablets with her on holiday and has missed several doses.

Question 97
Theme: The treatment of endocrine conditions

Options:

A	Desmopressin	J	Thyroxine
B	Calciferol	K	Octreotide
C	Intravenous calcium gluconate		
D	Phenoxybenzamine and propranolol		
E	Metyrapone		
F	Long-term replacement with glucocorticoids and mineralocorticoids		
G	Propranolol		
H	Carbimazole		
I	Propylthiouracil		

For each case below, choose the SINGLE most appropriate treatment from the above list of options. Each option may be used once, more than once, or not at all.

1. A 40-year-old man presents to his GP complaining of change in appearance and headaches. His brow is more prominent, and his nose has broadened. He states that his shoes are too small, and he has tingling in certain fingers worse at night.

2. A 50-year-old woman presents to her GP for fatigue, depression and weight gain. She also complains of constipation and poor memory. On examination, she has a smooth peaches and cream complexion, thin eyebrows, and a large tongue.

3. A 35-year-old pregnant woman presents to her GP with anxiety. On examination, she is a nervous woman with exophthalmos, warm peripheries, and atrial fibrillation.

4. A 50-year-old obese woman presents to Casualty with rib fractures and bruising following a fall in the loo. She is noted to be hypertensive and have glycosuria.

5. A 70-year-old woman presents to her GP with weight loss and depression. On examination, she is noted to have buccal pigmentation and pigmented scars. She appears dehydrated. Her BP is 100/60.

Question 98
Theme: Investigation of dermatological lesions

Options:

A	Skin scrapings	J	Chest X-ray
B	Skin biopsy	K	Kveim test
C	Wood's light	L	Mantoux test
D	Patch tests	M	ESR
E	Urine testing for glucose		
F	Full blood count		
G	Immunofluorescent staining of skin sample		
H	Antinuclear antibodies		
I	Clotting screen		

For each presentation below, choose the SINGLE most discriminating investigation from the above list of options. Each option may be used once, more than once, or not at all.

1. A 7-year-old girl presents with an itchy rash in her elbow creases and behind her knees. Lichenification is seen in both the elbow and knee flexures.

2. A 10-year-old boy presents with areas of scaling and hair loss. On examination, there are areas of crusting on the scalp and matting of the hair.

3. A 33-year-old female presents with a facial rash and a rash on the back of her hands. She is noted to have a maculopapular rash over her forehead, nose and cheeks and a blue-red discolouration of the back of her hands.

4. A 40-year-old man presents with areas of erythema and scaling of the skin of the groin and perianal region.

5. A 65-year-old man presents with irritation and erythema of the skin and blister formation. The blisters are over his legs and are tense.

Question 99
Theme: Diagnosis of vitamin deficiency

Options:

A Vitamin A deficiency	J Folic acid deficiency
B Vitamin D deficiency	K Cobalamin deficiency
C Vitamin K deficiency	L Ascorbic acid deficiency
D Vitamin E deficiency	
E Thiamine deficiency	
F Riboflavin deficiency	
G Niacin deficiency	
H Pyridoxine deficiency	
I Biotin deficiency	

For each presentation, choose the SINGLE most likely diagnosis from the above list of options. Each option may be used once, more than once, or not at all.

1. A 9-year-old boy is noted to have a Bitot spot on his conjunctiva.

2. A 40-year-old female with a history of coeliac disease presents with epistaxis. Her prothrombin time is elevated.

3. A 30-year-old man presents with fissuring of the angles of his mouth and seborrheic dermatitis around his nose.

4. A 40-year-old man complains of flushing after coffee and alcohol and diarrhoea. On examination, he has angular stomatitis, a Casal's collar rash, and oedema.

5. A 30-year-old woman presents to her dentist with bleeding gums. She does not like to eat vegetables.

Question 100
Theme: Causes of vertigo

Options:

A	Migraine	I	Arrhythmias
B	Vestibular neuronitis	J	Meniere's disease
C	Multiple sclerosis	K	Acoustic neuroma
D	Lateral medullary syndrome	L	Postural hypotension
E	Wernicke's encephalopathy		
F	Vertebrobasilar ischaemia		
G	Epilepsy		
H	Hypoglycaemia		

For each case below, choose the SINGLE most likely cause from the above list of options. Each option may be used once, more than once, or not at all.

1. A 40-year-old man presents with vertigo, nausea, and weakness. He also complains of tingling sensation down his right arm and of double vision in one eye. On examination, he has loss of central vision, nystagmus, and ataxia.

2. A 50-year-old man presents with severe vertigo with vomiting and left-sided facial pain. On examination, he has nystagmus on looking to the left. His soft palate is paralysed on the left side, and he has analgaesia to pinprick on the left side of the face and right limbs. He also has a left-sided Horner's syndrome.

3. A 50-year-old woman presents with vertigo and unilateral deafness. The attacks of vertigo last for hours and are accompanied by vomiting. On examination, she has nystagmus and a low frequency sensorineural hearing loss.

4. A 20-year-old man presents with sudden onset of vertigo and vomiting. He denies tinnitus or hearing loss. He had an upper respiratory tract infection a week prior.

5. A 60-year-old man presents with vertigo brought on by turning his head, ataxia, dysarthria, and nystagmus.

Question 101
Theme: Investigation of syncope

Options:

A	Serum glucose	J	Urinanalysis
B	12 lead electrocardiogram	K	Arterial blood gas
C	Chest X-ray	L	Blood cultures
D	Computerised tomography (CT scan) of the head		
E	Electroencephalogram		
F	Serum calcium		
G	Serum electrolytes and urea		
H	Full blood count		
I	Blood pressure readings when lying down and when standing		

For each case below, choose the SINGLE most discriminating investigation from the above list of options. Each option may be used once, more than once, or not at all.

1. A 50-year-old woman presents with a history of episodes of sudden weakness of the lower limbs and falling. There is no loss of consciousness.

2. A 60-year-old man presents with shaking, sweats, and fainting in the morning.

3. A 65-year-old woman with a history of chronic renal failure presents with fits and fainting. She complains of cramps in her limbs and circumoral numbness.

4. A 60-year-old woman complains of dizziness and blackouts. On examination, her pulse rate is 50.

5. A 70-year-old woman with Parkinson's disease on levodopa presents with fainting spells when getting up at night.

Question 102
Theme: Investigation of seizures

Options:

A	Serum calcium	J	Chest X-ray
B	Serum glucose	K	Drug levels
C	Serum electrolytes	L	Electroencephalogram
D	Serum urea and creatinine	M	ESR
E	Serum liver function tests	N	Anti-double-stranded
F	Full blood count		DNA
G	Computerised tomography (CT scan) of the head		
H	Lumbar puncture		
I	VDRL		

For each case below, choose the SINGLE most discriminating investigation from the above list of options. Each option may be used once, more than once, or not at all.

1. A 50-year-old alcoholic presents with sweating, tachycardia, and convulsions.

2. A 40-year-old diabetic started on tetracycline for severe aphthous ulceration now presents with epilepsy and vomiting.

3. A 10-year-old boy presents with fits for the first time. His parents report that he stops talking in mid sentence and then continues where he left off 10 seconds later.

4. A 15-year-old female presents with fits and fever. She is noted to have a petechial rash that does not blanch on pressure.

5. A 30-year-old woman presents with fits and arthralgia. She is noted to have thinning of her hair and oral ulceration.

Question 103
Theme: The treatment of respiratory diseases

Options:

A	Beta-2-adrenoreceptor agonist	J	Plasmapharesis
B	Intravenous aminophylline	K	Tetracycline
C	Erythromycin		
D	Tobramycin and carbenicillin		
E	Ciprofloxacin		
F	Co-trimoxazole		
G	Rifampicin and isoniazid		
H	Prednisolone		
I	Cyclophosphamide		

For each presentation below, choose the SINGLE most appropriate treatment from the above list of options. Each option may be used once, more than once, or not at all.

1. A 12-year-old boy with cystic fibrosis presents with a chest infection. The boy also suffers from mild renal failure.

2. A 40-year-old mental patient presents with dry cough and confusion. Blood tests reveal lymphopaenia and hyponatraemia. Chest X-ray shows right-sided lobar shadowing.

3. A 10-year-old boy presents with wheezing attacks and episodic shortness of breath. His peak expiratory flow rate is 400 L/min.

4. A 40-year-old male presents with rhinorrhea, cough, haemoptysis, and pleuritic pain. Chest X-ray shows multiple nodules.

5. A 60-year-old farmer presents with fever, cough, and shortness of breath. He had been forking hay that morning. Chest X-ray shows fluffy nodular shadows in the upper zones.

Question 104
Theme: The treatment of facial pain

Options:

A	Prednisolone	J	Augmentin and nasal decongestant
B	Tricyclic antidepressant	K	Analgesia
C	Lithium carbonate		
D	Broad-spectrum antibiotics		
E	Ergotamine		
F	Serotonin antagonist		
G	Propranolol		
H	Carbamazepine		
I	Refer patient to dentist		

For each case below, choose the SINGLE most appropriate treatment from the above list of options. Each option may be used once, more than once, or not at all.

1. A 30-year-old woman presents with unilateral headache and facial pain. She describes flashing lights preceding the headache and nausea. She is asthmatic and is on the oral contraceptive pill. She also suffers from Grave's disease.

2. A 40-year-old man complains of a series of headaches that occur every year and consist of severe pain around the eye for 3 weeks at a time.

3. A 35-year-old woman complains of frontal headaches and pain over the bridge of her nose with catarrh and nasal blockage.

4. A 55-year-old woman complains of pain in her face and jaw worse on eating. She also complains of transient loss of vision in her right eye and scalp pain when combing her hair.

5. A 50-year-old woman complains of an electric shock-like pain that starts in her jaw and ascends to her temples. She states the pain is agonising and is triggered by touching a particular spot on her lips.

Question 105
Theme: Diagnosis of peripheral nerve injuries

Options:

A	Erb's palsy	I	Suprascapular nerve injury
B	Klumpke's palsy		
C	Long thoracic nerve injury	J	Sciatic nerve injury
D	Spinal accessory nerve injury	K	Femoral nerve injury
E	Axillary nerve injury	L	Tibial nerve injury
F	Radial nerve injury	M	Common peroneal nerve injury
G	Ulnar nerve injury		
H	Median nerve injury	N	Superficial peroneal nerve injury

For each patient below, choose the SINGLE most likely diagnosis from the above list of options. Each option may be used once, more than once, or not at all.

1. A football player presents with a drop foot after injuring his knee. He can neither dorsiflex nor evert the foot. Sensation is lost over the front and outer half of the leg and dorsum of the foot.

2. A 50-year-old man post incision and drainage of a posterior triangle neck abscess now presents with pain and drooping of his shoulder. On examination, there is mild winging of the scapula on active abduction of the arm against resistance. This then disappears on forward thrusting of the shoulder.

3. A 20-year-old man who has accidently cut his forearm on shattered glass now presents with hyperextension of the meta-carpophalangeal joints of the ring and little fingers.

4. A 30-year-old man presents with an elbow dislocation and a hand held with the ulnar fingers flexed and the index straight. He is unable to abduct his thumb.

5. A 60-year-old man post total hip replacement now walks with a drop foot and a high-stepping gait. Sensation is lost below the knees except over the medial leg.

Question 106
Theme: Diagnosis of back pain

Options:

A	Discitis	J	Osteoarthritis
B	Proplased lumbar disc	K	Scoliosis
C	Senile kyphosis		
D	Tuberculosis		
E	Pyogenic spondylitis		
F	Adolescent kyphosis (Scheuermann's disease)		
G	Lumbar spondylosis		
H	Spinal stenosis		
I	Spondylolisthesis		

For each patient below, choose the SINGLE most likely diagnosis from the above list of options. Each option may be used once, more than once, or not at all.

1. A 30-year-old female presents with back pain and pain in the buttock and lower limb. She was moving house and lifting heavy objects. She stands with a slight list to one side. Straight leg raise is restricted and painful.

2. A 60-year-old man presents with longstanding back pain and ill-health. On examination, he has a hunchback. The X-ray shows destruction of the front of the vertebral bodies and calcification of a psoas abscess.

3. A 13-year-old female presents with a convexity of 70 degrees in her thoracic spine.

4. A 12-year-old female presents with backache and fatigue. On examination, she has rounded shoulders with a hump and a lumbar lordosis.

5. A 50-year-old female presents with chronic backache. On examination, the buttocks are flat, the sacrum appears to extend to the waist, and the transverse loin creases are seen. A step can be felt when the fingers are run down the spine.

Question 107
Theme: Diagnosis of limp in childhood

Options:

A	Congenital dislocation of the hip	I	Tuberculosis
B	Perthes' disease	J	Coxa vara
C	Slipped epiphysis	K	Irritable hip
D	Tumour	L	Pyogenic arthritis
E	Avascular necrosis		
F	Acquired dislocation of the hip		
G	Femoral anteversion		
H	Acetabular dysplasia and subluxation of the hip		

For each case below, choose the SINGLE most likely diagnosis from the above list of options. Each option may be used once, more than once, or not at all.

1. A 6-week-old girl is examined and abduction of the hip is found to be impeded, but with pressure applied to the greater trochanter, the hip is able to abduct fully.

2. A 6-year-old girl presents with a painful hip after exercise. On examination, she has a positive Trendelenburg sign, asymmetrical leg lengths, and the femoral head is palpated as a lump in the groin. Abduction is limited.

3. A 1-year-old boy presents with a limp. The leg is short, and the thigh is bowed. His femoral-neck shaft angle is 110 degrees.

4. A 15-year-old boy presents with a left leg limp and pain in the groin. On examination, the leg is turned out and 2 cm shorter than the right leg. There is limitation of flexion, abduction, and medial rotation. As the hip is flexed, there is increased external rotation.

5. A 7-year-old boy presents with a right leg limp and pain in the groin. Extremes of all movements are limited. He has had a similar episode 6 months ago that resolved spontaneously.

Question 108
Theme: Diagnosis of ankle and foot deformities

Options:

A	Hallux rigidus	I	Osteoarthritis
B	Hallux valgus	J	Ruptured tendo Achilles
C	Pes cavus	K	Diabetic foot
D	Hammer toe	L	Gout
E	Mallet toe	M	Plantar fasciitis
F	Rheumatoid arthritis		
G	Morton's metatarsalgia		
H	Stress fracture		

For each presentation below, choose the SINGLE most likely diagnosis from the above list of options. Each option may be used once, more than once, or not at all.

1. A 45-year-old man complains that he is unable to tiptoe. He feels as though he has been struck above the heel. Plantarflexion is weak. With the patient prone, the foot remains still when the calf is squeezed.

2. A 60-year-old man is noted for bilateral foot deformities. He has swollen, painless feet, claw toes, and plantar ulceration over the metatarsal heads. He also has an amputated 5th toe digit.

3. A 50-year-old woman complains of sharp pain in the forefoot radiating to the toes. Tenderness is elicited in the third inter-digital space, and sensation is diminished in the cleft.

4. A 40-year-old woman presents with a second toe deformity. The proximal joint is fixed in flexion, and the metatarso-phalangeal joint is extended. She has a painful callous on the dorsum of the toe and under the metatarsal head.

5. A 50-year-old woman presents with pain on walking. On examination, the metatarsophalangeal joint is enlarged and tender, with a callosity under the medial side of the distal phalanx. Dorsiflexion is restricted and painful.

Question 109

Theme: Diagnosis of lower limb fractures

Options:

A	Pelvic fracture	I	Fracture of the proximal
B	Sacrococcygeal fracture		fibula
C	Femoral neck fracture	J	Fractured patella
D	Supracondylar fracture	K	Fractured tibial spine
E	Femoral condyle fracture		
F	Intertrochanteric fracture		
G	Tibial plateau fracture		
H	Femoral shaft fracture		

For each case below, choose the SINGLE most likely diagnosis from the above list of options. Each option may be used once, more than once, or not at all.

1. A 20-year-old cyclist was struck in a RTA and is brought into Casualty. His perineum and scrotum are swollen and bruised. He is unable to pass urine, and there is a streak of blood at the external meatus.

2. A 70-year-old woman catches her toe in the carpet and falls, twisting the hip into external rotation. On examination, her leg is in lateral rotation and appears short. She is able to take some steps.

3. An 80-year-old woman presents to Casualty after a fall directly onto her hip and is now unable to weight-bear. The leg is shorter and externally rotated. She cannot lift her leg.

4. A 20-year-old female was roller-blading when she fell. She is now unable to weight-bear. On examination, her leg is rotated externally and is shorter. The thigh is swollen and bruised.

5. A 10-year-old child twisted his knee and now presents with a swollen immobile knee. The joint is tense, tender and doughy. Aspiration reveals a haemarthrosis. Examination under anaesthesia shows that extension is blocked.

Question 110
Theme: The treatment of fractures and dislocations

Options:

A   Kocher's method
B   AO cannulated screws
C   Bedrest
D   Open reduction and Kirschner wire
E   Buddy strapping
F   Reconstructive surgery with internal graft or implant augmentation
G   Physiotherapy for strengthening exercises
H   Austin Moore hemiarthroplasty
I   Dynamic hip screw
J   Total hip replacement
K   Open reduction and internal fixation

For each of the cases below, choose the SINGLE most appropriate treatment from the above list of options. Each option may be used once, more than once, or not at all.

1. A 50-year-old fit man presents with a right hip fracture. On X-ray, the fracture line is sub-capital.

2. A 20-year-old athlete twists his knee on holiday while skiing. On examination, he has a positive drawer sign with the tibia sliding anteriorly.

3. A 70-year-old woman presents with a left hip fracture. On X-ray, the fracture line is intertrochanteric.

4. A 40-year-old woman sprains her wrist. She complains of persistent pain and tenderness over the dorsum distal to Lister's tubercle. X-rays show a large gap between the scaphoid and the lunate. In the lateral view, the lunate is tilted dorsally and the scaphoid anteriorly.

5. A 30-year-old basketball player presents with severe pain in his shoulder. He is holding his arm with the opposite hand. He explains that he fell on an outstretched hand. The X-ray shows overlapping shadows of the humeral head and glenoid fossa, with the head lying below and medial to the socket. There is also a fracture of the neck of the humerus.

Question 111
Theme: The treatment of upper limb injuries

Options:

A   Sling
B   Kocher's method
C   Collar and cuff
D   Open reduction and Kirschner
    wire fixation
E   Buddy strapping
F   Open reduction and internal
    fixation
G   Traction on the arm in
    abduction followed by rotation
    of the arm laterally with
    pressure on the humeral head

H   Closed reduction and
    cast immobilisation
I   Open reduction and
    plating
J   Plaster cast immobilisation
    alone
K   Splinting in a plaster cast

For each case below, choose the SINGLE most appropriate treatment from the above list of options. Each option may be used once, more than once, or not at all.

1. A 40-year-old man with a history of epilepsy presents with right shoulder pain. The arm is held in medial rotation with a flat shoulder. The anteroposterior film shows a humeral head like an electric light bulb and an empty glenoid sign.

2. An 8-year-old boy presents with a painful and swollen elbow. He fell onto his outstretched hand. The lateral X-ray shows an undisplaced supracondylar fracture line running obliquely downwards and forwards.

3. A 70-year-old female with osteoporosis falls onto the back of her hand. She presents with wrist pain. The X-ray shows a fracture through the distal radial metaphysis, and the distal fragment is displaced and tilted anteriorly.

4. A 3-year-old child presents with a painful, dangling arm after having her arm jerked. The forearm is held in pronation. There are no X-ray changes.

5. A 25-year-old man presents with a swollen, tender finger. X-ray shows a transverse, undisplaced fracture of the proximal phalanx.

Question 112
Theme: The treatment of back pain

Options:

A	Physiotherapy	I	Radiotherapy
B	Rest, weight loss, analgesia	J	Excision of the nidus
C	Surgical removal of a prolapsed disc		
D	Nerve root decompression		
E	Spinal decompression with laminectomy		
F	Lateral mass fusion		
G	Calcitonin		
H	Chemotherapy		

For each case below, choose the SINGLE most appropriate treatment from the above list of options. Each option may be used once, more than once, or not at all.

1. A 30-year-old man presents with bone pain around the knee. X-ray shows bony destruction and periosteal elevation with sub-periosteal new bone formation. Chest X-ray reveals nodules.

2. A 70-year-old man presents with low back pain, aching and numbness in his thighs and legs. He prefers to walk uphill than downhill. His activities are now severely restricted. X-ray reveals a trefoil-shaped lumbar spinal canal and osteoarthritic changes.

3. A 60-year-old man presents with chronic back pain. On examination he has a large head and bowed shins. He is hard of hearing. X-rays show sclerosis and osteoporosis. His blood tests show an elevated alkaline phosphatase.

4. A 70-year-old woman presents with chronic back pain. On examination, she is tender along her shoulders, ribs and back. Blood tests reveal a high calcium and a high urea. X-rays show osteolytic lesions.

5. A 20-year-old man presents with a painful shin. Aspirin seems to relieve the pain. On X-ray, there is a localised osteolytic lesion surrounded by a rim of sclerosis.

Question 113
Theme: The treatment of intestinal obstruction

Options:

A	Right hemicolectomy	H	Abdominoperineal resection with end colostomy
B	Urgent herniorrhaphy		
C	Sigmoid colectomy		
D	Nasogastric aspiration with fluid and electrolyte replacement	I	Transverse colectomy
E	Subtotal colectomy and ileorectal anastomosis	J	Proximal loop colostomy
F	Anterior resection		
G	Exploratory laparotomy and Hartmann's procedure		

For each presentation below, choose the SINGLE most appropriate treatment from the above list of options. Each option may be used once, more than once, or not at all.

1. A 60-year-old man presents with abdominal pain in the right iliac fossa and distension. X-ray shows a single dilated loop of bowel of 12 cm in diameter with the convexity under the left hemidiaphragm.

2. A 70-year-old man presents with bowel obstruction and pain in the rectum. Rectal exam and biopsy confirm an obstructing carcinoma of the rectum.

3. A 50-year-old man complains of constant groin pain, associated with nausea and vomiting. On examination, he has a positive cough impulse. A tender, tense lump is palpated and is not reducible.

4. A 60-year-old man presents with fever, vomiting, and intense left iliac fossa pain. On examination, he has a rigid, distended abdomen with rebound tenderness on the left. Erect chest X-ray reveals free air under the diaphragm.

5. An 80-year-old man presents with abdominal distension and pain. Sigmoidoscopy and barium enema confirm an obstructing carcinoma of the rectosigmoid.

Question 114
Theme: Causes of pain in the lower extremities

Options:

A Buerger's disease
B Varicose veins
C Leriche syndrome
D Femoral-popliteal disease
E Acute arterial occlusion of the lower limb
F Post-traumatic vasomotor dystrophy
G Raynaud's phenomenon
H Phlebitis
I Anterior tibial compartment syndrome
J Osteomyelitis
K Deep venous thrombosis

For each patient below, choose the SINGLE most likely cause from the above list of options. Each option may be used once, more than once, or not at all.

1. A 30-year-old marathan runner presents with intense pain in his anterolateral calf. On examination, he has a swollen leg with pain on dorsiflexion and numbness in the first dorsal web space.

2. A 50-year-old woman presents with pain in the calves after prolonged standing. On examination, she has mild ankle oedema, paper thin skin, an ulcer over the medial molleolus and lipodermatosclerosis.

3. A 60-year-old man with a history of myocardial infarction now presents with a painful left leg. On examination, the leg is cold. Peripheral pulses cannot be palpated. He cannot lift his leg and complains of pins and needles in the leg.

4. A 55-year-old man presents with buttock and thigh pain. He is impotent.

5. A 60-year-old man complains of pain in the calves, severe enough to limit his mobility. The pain is now in his feet and worse at night in bed. He hangs his leg over the side of the bed to relieve the pain. Buerger's test is positive.

Question 115
Theme: The treatment of dysphagia

Options:

A	Antifungal therapy	J	H2-receptor antagonists
B	Incision and drainage		
C	Endoscopic diverticulotomy		
D	External excision of pharyngeal pouch		
E	Reassurance		
F	Nasogastric intubation		
G	Intravenous antibiotics and analgesia		
H	Antispasmodics		
I	Dilatation of the lower oesophageal sphincter		

For each case below, choose the SINGLE most appropriate treatment from the above list of options. Each option may be used once, more than once, or not at all.

1. A 50-year-old man complains of dysphagia after eating bread. Barium swallow reveals a lower oesophageal ring.

2. A 40-year-old woman on chemotherapy for metastatic breast carcinoma now presents with painful swallowing. On examination, she has white plaques on top of friable mucosa in her mouth and more seen on oesophagoscopy.

3. A 20-year-old man presents with painful swallowing. On examination, he has trismus and unilateral enlargement of his tonsil. The peritonsillar region is red, inflamed and swollen.

4. A 40-year-old woman presents with dysphagia. On examination, she is febrile with neck erythema and a midline neck swelling.

5. A 40-year-old woman complains of dysphagia for both solids and liquids. She sometimes suffers from severe retrosternal chest pain. Barium swallow reveals a dilated oesophagus which tapers to a fine distal end.

Question 116
Theme: Diagnosis of genetic disorders and birth defects

Options:

A   Fetal alcohol syndrome
B   Fragile X syndrome
C   Marfan's syndrome
D   Trisomy 21
E   Turner's syndrome
F   Trisomy 13
G   Hurler syndrome

H   Homocystinuria
I   Phenylketonuria
J   Klinefelter's syndrome
K   Neurofibromatosis

For each patient below, choose the SINGLE most likely diagnosis from the above list of options. Each option may be used once, more than once, or not at all.

1. A 6-week-old infant presents with irritability. He is in the 2nd percentile for weight and length. On examination, he has a small midface and a long philtrum. He has clinodactyly of the fifth finger and cervical vertebral fusion.

2. An 8-year-old girl presents to her GP with scoliosis. She is in the 100th percentile for her height. She wears glasses for myopia and is of normal intelligence. On examination, she is noted to have a mid-systolic click and a late systolic murmur. She also has hypermobile joints.

3. A 10-year-old boy presents with chest pain and is diagnosed with acute myocardial infarction. He is tall with long limbs and digits. He has a dislocated lens and is mildly mentally retarded.

4. A 10-year-old boy presents with progressive mental retardation. He is in the 5th percentile for his height. He has a large head and coarse facies. He is noted to have hepatomegaly.

5. A 15-year-old girl presents to the GP as she has not started to menstruate and has no breast development. She is in the 3rd percentile for her height. She has learning difficulties at school. On examination, she has a mid-systolic ejection murmur on auscultation and multiple pigmented skin naevi.

Question 117
Theme: The treatment of airway obstruction

Options:

A	Nebulised salbutamol	J	Heimlich manoeuvre
B	Intramuscular adrenaline 1:1000	K	Suction of mucous plug
C	Endotracheal intubation	L	CPAP
D	Tracheostomy		
E	Hyperbaric oxygen		
F	Oxygen and adequate fluids		
G	Fibre-optic bronchoscopy		
H	Endotracheal intubation and intravenous ceftazidime		
I	Needle thoracocentesis		

For each presentation below, choose the SINGLE most appropriate treatment from the above list of options. Each option may be used once, more than once, or not at all.

1. A 15-year-old boy presents choking on a boiled sweet. He suddenly becomes quiet and turns blue.

2. A 15-year-old girl presents to Casualty after being stung by a wasp. She is acutely distressed and dyspnoeic. She develops stridor.

3. A 4-year-old boy presents with high fever and stridor. He is in severe respiratory distress. He is drooling saliva.

4. A 70-year-old woman with a tracheostomy tube now presents with difficulty breathing. She is apyrexial. She complains that her tube feels blocked.

5. A 60-year-old man with a history of chronic bronchitis presents with tachypnoea and wheezing throughout the chest.

Question 118
Theme: The treatment of neck lumps

Options:

A	Incision and drainage	J	Thyroid lobectomy
B	Intravenous antibiotics		
C	Sistrunk's operation		
D	Endoscopic diverticulotomy		
E	External excision		
F	Antituberculous chemotherapy		
G	Submandibular gland excision		
H	Total thyroidectomy		
I	Excisional biopsy		

For each case below, choose the SINGLE most appropriate treatment from the above list of options. Each option may be used once, more than once, or not at all.

1. A 20-year-old man presents with a mobile midline neck swelling that moves when he sticks out his tongue.

2. A 50-year-old man presents with a right neck swelling that is discharging malodorous cheesy discharge. Chest X-ray shows patchy shadows in the left apex.

3. A 30-year-old woman presents with a 4 cm cystic swelling over the anterior third of her left sternomastoid muscle.

4. A 40-year-old man presents with a midline neck swelling. The swelling has grown to 5 cm over 6 weeks and moves upon swallowing. Fine needle aspiration shows anaplastic cells.

5. A 60-year-old smoker presents with a 6 cm neck lump in the posterior triangle. The fine needle aspirate is inconclusive.

Question 119
Theme: Diagnosis of intracranial lesions

Options:

A	Subdural haematoma	I	Cerebral angioma
B	Cerebral abscess	J	Subarachnoid haemorrhage
C	Astrocytoma		
D	Acoustic neuroma	K	Extradural haematoma
E	Meningioma	L	Medulloblastoma
F	Pituitary tumour		
G	Secondary tumour		
H	Cerebral aneurysm		

For each case, choose the SINGLE most likely diagnosis from the above list of options. Each option may be used once, more than once, or not at all.

1. A 50-year-old man presents with unilateral tinnitus and dizziness. He also complains of difficulty swallowing and loss of taste.

2. A 45-year-old woman presents with sudden onset of headache, neck stiffness, and double vision. She lapses into a coma. She had a similar episode 2 weeks prior that was not as severe and resolved spontaneously. She has a history of hypertension and no history of head trauma.

3. A 10-year-old boy presents with headache, blurry vision, and vomiting. He is noted to have an ataxic gait, nystagmus and past pointing. His CT scan of the head shows enlarged cerebral ventricles and a cerebellar mass.

4. A 40-year-old woman post radical mastectomy now presents with sudden onset of severe headache and confusion. She is apyrexial and shows no signs of head trauma. The CT scan of the head shows a space-occupying lesion.

5. A 30-year-old cricketer presents in a coma. He had been struck by a cricket ball earlier that day and had been fine until now. On examination he has asymmetrical pupils.

Question 120
Theme: Investigation of haemoptysis

Options:

A	Full blood count (FBC)	I	Heaf test
B	Clotting studies	J	Urinanalysis
C	Bronchography	K	Pulmonary angiogram
D	Chest X-ray	L	Tissue biopsy
E	12 lead electrocardiogram	M	Sputum cytology
F	Antinuclear antibodies and free DNA		
G	Anti-glomerular basement antibody in the serum		
H	Computerised tomography of the chest		

For each case below, choose the SINGLE most discriminating investigation from the above list of options. Each option may be used once, more than once, or not at all.

1. A 40-year-old man presents with recurrent epistaxis, haemoptysis, and haematuria. On examination, he has a nasal septal perforation and nodules on chest X-ray.

2. A 30-year-old man presents with haemoptysis, dyspnoea and haematuria. Chest X-ray reveals bilateral alveolar infiltrates. Urinalysis reveals the presence of protein and red cell casts.

3. A 60-year-old man presents with a chronic cough and mild haemoptysis. On examination, he has digital clubbing with pain and swelling around his wrists. Chest X-ray reveals a single nodule.

4. A 30-year-old IVDA presents with dyspnoea and haemoptysis. His chest X-ray is unremarkable, and the ECG shows a sinus tachycardia with a mean P axis shift to the right. Blood gas shows a low PCO_2 and an elevated pH.

5. A 50-year-old man presents with occasional haemoptysis and chronic productive cough. He has a history of recurrent pneumonia. Chest X-ray reveals peribronchial fibrosis.

Question 121
Theme: Causes of proteinuria

Options:

A	Alport's syndrome	I	Diabetic nephropathy
B	Minimal change disease	J	Henoch-Schönlein
C	Lupus nephritis		purpura
D	Focal glomerulosclerosis	K	Goodpasture's
E	Membranoproliferative		syndrome
	glomerulonephritis	L	Postinfectious
F	Mesangial proliferative		glomerulonephritis
	glomerulonephritis		
G	Membranous glomerulonephritis		
H	Idiopathic crescenteric		
	glomerulonephritis		

For each case below, choose the SINGLE most likely cause from the above list of options. Each option may be used once, more than once, or not at all.

1. A 40-year-old man presents with proteinuria, haematuria, and progressive renal failure. He is noted to have a high frequency sensorineural hearing loss. He has a sister who was noted to have microscopic haematuria but is asymptomatic.

2. A 7-year-old boy presents with generalised oedema and proteinuria. Electron microscopy reveals fusion of the epithelial foot processes and normal appearing capillary and basement membranes.

3. A 30-year-old heroin addict presents with hypertension, oedema, oliguria, and is noted to have heavy proteinuria. Renal biopsy specimen reveals loss of glomerular cellularity and collapse of capillary loops. Adhesions between portions of the glomerular tuft and Bowman's capsule are also seen.

4. A 12-year-old boy presents with sudden onset of haematuria and oedema. Further investigations reveal proteinuria and hypocomplementaemia (C3). Sub-epithelial humps and foot process fusion are seen by electron microscopy.

5. A 4-year-old boy presents with a faint leg rash, bloody diarrhoea, and oliguria. Further investigations reveal heavy proteinuria and an elevated serum IgA.

Question 122
Theme: Causes of sexually transmitted diseases

Options:

A	Gardnerella	I	Phthrius pubis
B	*Neisseria gonorrhoeae*	J	*Trichomonas vaginalis*
C	Herpes simplex virus	K	*Candida albicans*
D	*Treponema pallidum*		
E	*Haemophilus ducreyi*		
F	*Calymmatobacterium granulomatis*		
G	*Chlamydia trachomatis*		
H	Human papilloma virus		

For each presentation below, choose the SINGLE most likely cause from the above list of options. Each option may be used once, more than once, or not at all.

1. A 28-year-old homosexual man presents with proctalgia and bloody anal discharge. Gram-staining of the anal discharge shows Gram-negative intracellular diplococci.

2. A 30-year-old man presents with large groin nodes and a penile ulcer. On examination there are nodes present on either side of the inguinal ligament and a vesicle on his penis.

3. A 30-year-old man presents with painless genital ulcers. The ulcers have rolled edges. Scrapings demonstrate Donovan bodies with Giemsa staining.

4. A 20-year-old man presents with multiple painful genital ulcers and suppurative inguinal nodes. The edges of the ulcers are ragged and undermined.

5. A 30-year-old woman presents with a solitary, painless genital ulcer with a hard, indurated base. Dark ground microscopy of the chancre fluid is diagnostic.

Question 123
Theme: Causes of bacterial infections

Options:

A Bacillus anthracis
B Pseudomonas pyocaneus
C Streptococcus pyogenes
D Staphylococcus aureus
E Corynebacterium diphtheriae
F Listeria monocytogenes
G Clostridum perfringens
H Borrelia burgdorferi

I Pseudomonas aeruginosa
J Escherichia coli
K Bordetella pertussis
L Yersinia enterocolitica
M Moraxella catarrhalis

For each case below, choose the SINGLE most likely causative organism from the above list of options. Each option may be used once, more than once, or not at all.

1. A 50-year-old diabetic complains of severe otalgia. On examination, there is granulation tissue present in the ear canal.

2. A 20-year-old man presents with fever, rash, and is unable to close his left eye. On examination, he is noted to have a skin rash with central clearing spreading from a tick bite and a left-sided facial palsy.

3. A 50-year-old alcoholic with known liver disease presents with fever, abdominal pain and distention. Paracentesis of the peritoneal fluid with Gram staining reveals Gram-negative rods.

4. A 55-year-old abattoir worker presents with fever, oedema, and a cutaneous pustule. Scraping of the skin lesion reveal Gram-positive rods.

5. A 60-year-old IDDM male presents with a painful and swollen leg. X-ray of the leg reveals air in the soft tissues.

Question 124
Theme: Causes of amenorrhoea

Options:

A	Prolactinoma	I	Ovarian failure
B	Stein–Leventhal syndrome	J	Drugs causing
C	Hypothyroidism		hyperprolactinaemia
D	Cushing's syndrome	K	Anorexia
E	Exercise-induced		
F	Kallman's syndrome		
G	Gonadal tumour		
H	Imperforate hymen		

For each patient below, choose the SINGLE most likely cause from the above list of options. Each option may be used once, more than once, or not at all.

1. A 20-year-old obese woman presents to the GP with amenorrhoea. She is noted to be hirsute and have severe acne. She gives a history of ovarian cysts.

2. A 16-year-old woman presents to the GP with primary amenorrhoea. She also complains of lack of smell and is noted to be colour-blind. Investigations reveal a low FSH.

3. A 20-year-old woman presents with galactorrhoea and amenorrhoea. Her urine pregnancy test is negative. She takes cimetidine for dyspepsia. Her serum prolactin level is 2000 mu/L.

4. A 30-year-old obese hirsute woman presents with amenorrhoea. Her blood pressure is 170/90, and her urine dipstick is positive for glucose.

5. A 25-year-old petite ballet dancer presents with amenorrhoea. She is wearing several layers of clothing. She explains that she is sensitive to the cold. On examination, she has lanugo.

Question 125
Theme: Investigation of rheumatic diseases

Options:

A	HLA B27 antigen	I	Anti-centromere antibody
B	Bone scan		
C	Antibody to ds DNA	J	Anti-Jo-1 antibody
D	Anti-nucleolus antibody	K	Serum uric acid
E	Rheumatoid factor	L	Anti-Ro antibody
F	HLA-DR4 antigen		
G	Synovial fluid analysis with polarised-light microscopy		
H	X-ray		

For each case below, choose the SINGLE most discriminating investigation from the above list of options. Each option may be used once, more than once, or not at all.

1. A 60-year-old alcoholic man presents with a hot, swollen first metatarsophalangeal joint and a lesion on the rim of his left pinna.

2. A 65-year-old woman with a history of hypothyroidism presents with a warm, painful swollen knee with effusion. The serum calcium is normal. X-ray reveals chondrocalcinosis.

3. A 40-year-old woman presents with flexion deformities of her fingers. She has soft-tissue swelling of her digits. She also complains of difficulty swallowing and is noted to have a beaked nose and facial telangiectasia.

4. A 30-year-old woman presents with painful digits worse in the cold and difficulty swallowing. She is noted to have tapered fingers and a fixed facial expression with facial telangiectasia. X-ray reveals calcium around her fingers.

5. A 20-year-old woman presents with dry eyes, arthralgia, dysphagia, and Raynaud's phenomenon.

Question 126
Theme: Risk factors for oncological diseases

Options:

A	Nasopharyngeal carcinoma	J	Hodgkin's disease
B	Colorectal carcinoma	K	Oesophageal carcinoma
C	Non-Hodgkin's lymphoma		
D	Sinonasal tumours		
E	Gastric carcinoma		
F	Lung carcinoma		
G	Salivary gland carcinoma		
H	Carcinoma of the pancreas		
I	Thyroid carcinoma		

For each case below, choose the SINGLE most likely associated carcinoma from the above list of options. Each option may be used once, more than once, or not at all.

1. A 50-year-old man of Southern Chinese origin presents with unilateral conductive hearing loss. He is noted to have the Epstein–Barr virus.

2. A 40-year-old woman with Sjögren's disease now presents with painless neck nodes.

3. A 50-year-old woman with blood group A and a history of pernicious anaemia now presents with weight loss and epigastric discomfort.

4. A 40-year-old man of Northern Chinese origin presents with hoarseness and dysphagia. He has a prior history of suicidal attempt with lye ingestion.

5. A 70-year-old woman presents with stridor and a neck mass. She has a prior history of radiation to the neck as a child.

Question 127
Theme: Causes of diarrhoea

Options:

A	Campylobacter infection	J	Salmonellosis
B	Viral gastroenteritis	K	Irritable bowel
C	Ulcerative colitis		syndrome
D	Crohn's disease	L	*Clostridium perfringens*
E	Laxative abuse		infection
F	*Pseudomembranous colitis*	M	*Escherichia coli* infection
G	Shigella infection		
H	Cryptosporidiosis infection		

For each presentation below, choose the SINGLE most likely cause from the above list of options. Each option may be used once, more than once, or not at all.

1. A 30-year-old man with AIDS presents with profuse watery diarrhoea. Oocysts are detected in the stool.

2. A 25-year-old man presents with fever, bloody diarrhoea, and cramping for several weeks that does not resolve with antibiotic therapy. Proctosigmoidoscopy reveals red, raw mucosa and pseudopolyps.

3. A 60-year-old man presents with fever, watery diarrhoea and crampy abdominal pain. He had completed antibiotic therapy for osteomyelitis a month ago. Proctosigmoidoscopy reveals yellowish-white plaques on the mucosa.

4. A 20-year-old man recently back from holiday in the Far East presents with abrupt onset of severe diarrhoea. The diarrhoea is self-limiting and lasts only 3 days.

5. A 20-year-old female presents with chronic watery diarrhoea. She is emaciated. Stool electrolyte studies show an osmotic gap. Blood tests reveal hypokalaemia.

Question 128
Theme: Noninfectious causes of diarrhoea

Options:

A	Glucagonoma	
B	Coeliac disease	
C	Adenocarcinoma of the pancreas	
D	Colorectal carcinoma	
E	Crohn's disease	
F	Ulcerative colitis	
G	Thyrotoxicosis	
H	Diabetic neuropathy	
I	Faecal impaction	

J Metastatic carcinoid syndrome
K Zollinger–Ellison syndrome

For each patient below, choose the SINGLE most likely cause from the above list of options. Each option may be used once, more than once, or not at all.

1. A 40-year-old man presents with epigastric pain and diarrhoea. The basal gastric acid output rate is high.

2. A 50-year-old diabetic woman presents with weight loss, anaemia, and diarrhoea. She is noted to have migratory necrolytic erythema.

3. A 40-year-old woman presents with diarrhoea and weight loss. Small bowel biopsy reveals villous atrophy.

4. A 40-year-old man presents with weight loss and chronic diarrhoea. He is noted to have osteomas and colonic polyps.

5. A 20-year-old female presents with fever, weight loss, and diarrhoea. She is noted to have perianal fistulae. X-ray reveals a string sign.

Question 129
Theme: Diagnosis of haematological diseases

Options:

A Acute lymphoblastic leukaemia
B Multiple myeloma
C Acute myeloid leukaemia
D Idiopathic thrombocytopaenic purpura
E Chronic lymphocytic leukaemia
F Thrombotic thrombocytopaenic purpura
G Chronic myeloid leukaemia
H Polycythaemia rubra vera
I Amyloidosis
J Aplastic anaemia
K Primary myelosclerosis

For each case below, choose the SINGLE most likely diagnosis from the above list of options. Each option may be used once, more than once, or not at all.

1. A 70-year-old woman presents to her GP with weakness and bone pain. She also complains of blurry vision. She is noted to be anaemic with increased calcium and uric acid levels. X-ray reveals osteolytic bone lesions.

2. A 4-year-old boy presents with bone pain and weakness. Investigations reveal a pancytopaenia and blasts.

3. A 60-year-old man presents with malaise. He is noted to have gum hypertrophy and skin nodules. Investigations reveal a pancytopaenia and blasts.

4. A 50-year-old man presents with epistaxis. On examination, he has enlarged nontender neck nodes. His blood count reveals a lymphocytosis, anaemia and thrombocytopaenia.

5. A 40-year-old man presents with fever, sweats, and weight loss. He also suffers from gout. On examination, he has an enlarged spleen. Blood tests reveal a lymphocytosis and anaemia. The Philadelphia chromosome is detected.

Question 130
Theme: Investigations of skin lesions

Options:

A	Full blood count	I	Anti-Ro antibodies
B	Kveim test	J	Serum pancreatic
C	ANCA		glucagon
D	ESR	K	Muscle biopsy
E	Antibodies to double-stranded	L	Serum glucose
	DNA		
F	Skin biopsy		
G	Skin biopsy for Ziehl-Neelsen		
	staining for acid-fast bacilli		
H	Fasting cholesterol and		
	triglyceride levels		

For each presentation below, choose the SINGLE most discriminating investigation from the above list of options. Each option may be used once, more than once, or not at all.

1. A 38-year-old man presents with malaise and arthralgia. He is noted to have various skin lesions, including a purple bulbous nose and tender red raised nodules on his anterior shin.

2. A 70-year-old woman presents with a mid-facial disfigurement. The nose appears to have been gnawed off by a condition. The cutaneous lesion shows granulomas with central caseation.

3. A 50-year-old woman presents with fleshy-coloured papules over her right distal interphalangeal joint of her thumb and with a brown waxy plaque over her right shin.

4. A 50-year-old woman presents with weakness in her upper arms. She has difficulty combing her hair. On examination, she is noted to have ragged cuticles and nail fold capillary dilatation.

5. A 60-year-old woman presents with crops of yellow papules on her elbows and knees. Her serum glucose is normal.

Question 131
Theme: The treatment of medical emergencies

Options:

A	Intramuscular adrenaline	I	Intravenous dexamethasone
B	Emergency tracheostomy		
C	Urgent endotracheal intubation	J	Oxygen and nebulised salbutamol
D	Type and crossmatch blood		
E	Transfuse O negative blood and apply external fixator	K	Take patient straight to theatre
F	Transfer to burn unit		
G	Tetanus prophylaxis		
H	Intravenous antibiotics		

For each case below, choose the SINGLE most appropriate treatment from the above list of options. Each option may be used once, more than once, or not at all.

1. A 40-year-old pedestrian has been struck by a speeding car. She is brought into Accident and Emergency wearing a pneumatic antishock garment for an extensive open avulsion injury to her pelvis. She is intubated with fluids running via two large bore intravenous cannulas. Her blood pressure is 120/60. The pelvis is grossly distorted.

2. A 10-year-old boy burn victim is brought into Casualty with worsening stridor. A face mask with 100% oxygen is covering his face, but his oxygen saturation continues to fall. His mid-face and mouth have been severely burned.

3. A 4-year-old girl presents with fever, stridor and dyspnoea. She is sitting forward, drooling saliva. She has no history of asthma. She is becoming more distressed.

4. An 18-year-old man presents with fever, trismus and stridor. His breathing becomes laboured with use of accessory muscles. He becomes cyanotic. He initially presented to his GP with a sore throat a few days ago.

5. A 13-year-old known asthmatic presents with severe wheezing and a respiratory rate of 30. Her pulse rate is 120.

Question 132
Theme: Choices of contraception

Options:

A	Oral contraceptive	J	Barrier contraception
B	Condom and oral contraceptive		
C	IUCD		
D	Rhythm		
E	Bilateral tubal ligation		
F	Vasectomy		
G	The morning after pill		
H	Injectable contraceptive		
I	Douching		

For each patient below, choose the SINGLE most appropriate means of contraception from the above list of options. Each option may be used once, more than once, or not at all.

1. An 18-year-old university student would like to start having sexual relationships.

2. A 25-year-old woman living with her boyfriend asks advice regarding contraception.

3. A married 26-year-old healthy nulliparous woman would like to postpone having a family for 2 years.

4. A married 36-year-old obese mother of three with varicose veins and a 20 cigarette per day smoking habit would like a form of contraception.

5. A married 25-year-old woman with recent glandular fever would like a form of contraception as she would like to postpone starting a family for 1 year.

Question 133
Theme: The management of labour and delivery

Options:

A   Low transverse Caesarian section
B   Classic Caesarian section
C   Midforceps rotation
D   Syntocinon IV
E   Admit and perform external cephalic version daily
F   Spontaneous labour with vaginal delivery
G   External cephalic version in clinic
H   Intrauterine injection of prostaglandin F2α

I   Epidural anaesthesia
J   Episiotomy
K   Vacuum suction delivery
L   Hysterectomy

For each presentation below, choose the SINGLE most appropriate management from the above list of options. Each option may be used once, more than once, or not at all.

1. A 20-year-old nulliparous woman continues to bleed heavily following delivery of the baby and an intact placenta. Massaging the uterus, infusing IV syntocinon, and infusing blood fail to stem this postpartum haemorrhage.

2. A 25-year-old multiparous woman is found to carry a fetus with face presentation. There are no signs of fetal distress.

3. A 35-year-old multiparous woman of 39 weeks gestation is found to have a fetus in transverse lie presentation confirmed by ultrasound examination.

4. A 5′ 0″ nulliparous woman has prolonged labour lasting 20 hours. On examination, her cervix is dilated to 8 cm and the vertex is at −1 station. There have been no changes in the past 2 hours. She is still having regular contractions.

5. A 30-year-old primigravid has prolonged labour lasting 18 hours. The cervix is dilated to 8 cm. Fetal monitoring now shows late delecerations and a scalp pH of 7.2.

Question 134
Theme: Diagnosis of personality disorders

Options:

A	Schizoid	I	Antisocial
B	Borderline	J	Schizotypal
C	Narcissistic	K	Paranoid
D	Avoidant		
E	Passive-aggressive		
F	Obsessive-compulsive		
G	Multiple personality		
H	Histrionic		

For each patient below, choose the SINGLE most likely diagnosis from the above list of options. Each option may be used once, more than once, or not at all.

1. A 25-year-old man has no close friends. He avoids social situations. He is unable to express tender emotions. He has no overt signs of hallucination or delusional behaviour.

2. A 17-year-old boy is brought to his GP by his parents for abusive behaviour. He is delinquent from school and has been arrested for assault and for theft.

3. A 23-year-old man believes he is perfect. He is unable to empathise and manipulates people and situations. He sees everyone else as flawed. His relationships are shallow.

4. A 33-year-old female presents to the GP with chronic feelings of boredom and depression. She shops excessively and is sexually promiscuous. She has cut herself in the past to relieve her anxiety.

5. A 25-year-old anxious female presents to her GP. She suffers from low self-esteem and does not take risks in life. She seems extremely sensitive to criticism.

Question 135
Theme: Diagnosis of organic mental disorders

Options:

A   Parkinson's disease
B   Huntington's disease
C   Alzheimer's disease
D   Multi-infarct dementia
E   Creutzfeldt–Jakob disease
F   Korsakoff's psychosis
G   Temporal lobe seizures
H   Wernicke's encephalopathy
I   Chronic subdural haematoma
J   Subarachnoid haemorrhage
K   Acute intermittent porphyria

For each patient below, choose the SINGLE most likely diagnosis from the above list of options. Each option may be used once, more than once, or not at all.

1. A 70-year-old man presents with gradual deterioration of memory and intellect. His family have noticed a change in personality and behaviour.

2. A 35-year-old man presents with dementia and choreiform movements.

3. A 60-year-old alcoholic man presents with deterioration of both retrograde and anterograde memory. He invents stories.

4. A 60-year-old alcoholic man presents with persistent headache. His family notes that he is inattentive and becoming more confused. He had a fall a month ago.

5. A 65-year-old man presents with an abrupt onset of confusion and ataxia. On examination, he also has nystagmus. He is a known drinker.

Question 136
Theme: Diagnosis of psychiatric disorders

Options:

A	Schizophrenia	I	Delusional disorder
B	Brief reactive psychosis	J	Paranoid schizophrenia
C	Bipolar disorder	K	Postpartum depression
D	Major depression	L	Dysthymia
E	Body dysmorphic disorder		
F	Panic disorder		
G	Post-traumatic stress disorder		
H	Schizoaffective disorder		

For each patient below, choose the SINGLE most likely diagnosis from the above list of options. Each option may be used once, more than once or not at all.

1. A 40-year-old man insists that his wife is unfaithful and sleeping with the entire neighbourhood. He is hypersensitive, argumentative, and litiginous. His wife has left him due to his behaviour. He functions well at work.

2. A 25-year-old woman presents with personality changes. She is noted by friends initially to be anxious, irritable, and an insomniac and weeks later, she becomes profoundly depressed with low self-esteem and contemplates suicide. In consultation, she has pressured speech with boundless energy.

3. A 20-year-old woman has a 'mental breakdown'. She has recently broken up with her boyfriend. She has dramatic mood swings, memory loss, and incoherent speech. This lasts for a month.

4. A 20-year-old woman presents to her GP complaining of feeling depressed ever since she can remember. Her parents died in a car crash 10 years ago. She sees herself as a failure but functions well at work. She has trouble falling asleep.

5. A 50-year-old woman complains of sudden episodes of feeling impending doom. During these episodes she feels choked and sweats profusely.

Question 137
Theme: Diagnosis of childhood respiratory diseases

Options:

A   Bronchiolitis
B   Croup
C   Asthma
D   Cystic fibrosis
E   Epiglottitis
F   Obstructive sleep apnoea
G   *Chlamydia trachomatis* infection
H   Pneumonia
I   Allergic rhinitis

I   Influenza
J   Retrotonsillar abscess
K   Gonorrhoeal infection

For each patient below, choose the SINGLE most likely diagnosis from the above list of options. Each option may be used once, more than once, or not at all.

1. A 2-year-old boy presents with coughing and wheezing. Other members of the family are also suffering from an upper respiratory tract infection. On examination, he has flaring of the nostrils and audible expiratory wheezes.

2. A 10-year-old thin boy presents with chronic cough. Chest X-ray reveals bronchiectasis. He also suffers from steatorrhoea.

3. A 4-year-old boy presents to the GP for night terrors and loud snoring. On examination, he is a mouth breather with large tonsils that meet at the midline.

4. A 2-week-old infant presents with staccato cough and purulent conjunctivitis. On examination, he is apyrexial with diffuse rales on auscultation of the chest.

5. A 2-year-old boy presents with a 3-day history of noisy breathing on inspiration and a barking cough worse at night. He has a low grade fever and is hoarse.

Question 138
Theme: Causes of defects in the newborn from maternal infections

Options:

A	Hepatitis B	J	Group B streptococcus
B	Rubella	K	Group B coxsackie virus
C	Cytomegalovirus		
D	Toxoplasmosis		
E	Rubeola		
F	Varicella zoster		
G	Listeria		
H	*Neisseria gonorrhoea*		
I	*Chlamydia trachomatis*		

For each case below, choose the SINGLE most likely cause from the above list of options. Each option may be used once, more than once, or not at all.

1. A newborn baby is born with cataracts, cardiac defects, and deafness.

2. A newborn is noted to have microcephaly, epileptic fits, and chorioretinitis.

3. A stillbirth is also noted to have microcephaly and hepatosplenomegaly, and jaundice.

4. A newborn is noted to have eye abnormalities, skin scarring, and limb hypoplasia.

5. A newborn develops fatal encephalomyocarditis.

Question 139
Theme: Causes of genital tract bleeding in early pregnancy

Options:

A	Inevitable abortion	J	Cancer of the cervix
B	Missed abortion	K	Ectopic pregnancy
C	Complete abortion	L	Cervical erosion
D	Threatened abortion		
E	Incomplete abortion		
F	Hydatidiform mole		
G	Habitual abortion		
H	Cervical polyp		

For each case below, choose the SINGLE most likely cause from the above list of options. Each option may be used once, more than once, or not at all.

1. A nulliparous woman of 10 weeks gestation presents with uterine bleeding and pain. The internal os is open. There has been no passage of products of conception.

2. A primigravid of 8 weeks gestation presents with painless uterine bleeding. The serum and urinary hCG levels are much higher than expected for her gestation.

3. A primigravid of 20 weeks gestation has a small uterus that is not consistent with her last menstrual period date. She has not had uterine bleeding since the absence of fetal heart sounds 5 weeks ago.

4. A multiparous woman of 9 weeks gestation presents with uterine bleeding. The internal os is not dilated. The cervix is normal.

5. A primigravid of 10 weeks gestation presents wth uterine bleeding and passage of products of conception. The cervical os remains open.

Question 140
Theme: Diagnosis of thyroid diseases

Options:

A	Thyroglossal cyst	I	Simple goitre
B	Lingual thyroid	J	Follicular adenoma
C	Hashimoto's thyroiditis	K	deQuervain's thyroiditis
D	Riedel's thyroiditis	L	Acute thyroiditis
E	Graves' disease	M	Thyroid storm
F	Multinodular goitre		
G	Thyroid carcinoma		
H	Toxic multinodular goitre		

For each case below, choose the SINGLE most likely diagnosis from the above list of options. Each option may be used once, more than once, or not at all.

1. A 16-year-old girl presents with an anterior neck mass. It moves upward upon protrusion of her tongue. Thyroid radionucleotide scan shows no uptake in the midline.

2. A 40-year-old woman presents with a hard nodular midline neck mass. Blood tests reveal the presence of antibodies to thyroglobulin.

3. A 45-year-old woman presents with a diffuse swelling of the thyroid gland. On examination, she has a stare, lid lag, and lid retraction. On the dorsum of her legs she has areas of raised, peau d'orange-like, thickened skin. Blood tests reveal thyroid stimulating immunoglobulins against the TSH receptor site.

4. A 50-year-old woman presents with fever, tachycardia, restlessness, hypotension and vomiting. On examination, she has diffuse swelling of the thyroid gland and strabismus with diplopia.

5. A 35-year-old man presents with a hard, nodular midline neck mass that moves upward on deglutition. Thyroid radio-nucleotide scan shows cold spots.

Question 141
Theme: The management of traumatic injuries

Options:

A Peritoneal lavage
B Observation and angiography
C Closed thoracostomy-tube drainage
D Pressure dressing
E Cricothyroidotomy
F Nasogastric tube suction and observation
G Surgical repair of the flexor digitorum superficialis tendon

H Surgical repair of the flexor digitorum profundus tendon
I Urgent surgical exploration
J Debridement and repair
K Endotracheal intubation
L Needle pericardio-centesis
M Fasciotomy

For each case below, choose the SINGLE most appropriate management from the above list of options. Each option may be used once, more than once, or not at all.

1. A 23-year-old man presents to Accident and Emergency having been stabbed in the neck. He complains of difficulty swallowing and talking. He has no stridor. On examination, there is a small penetrating wound with diffuse neck swelling.

2. A 12-year-old boy presents with a hand injury sustained while playing rugby and attempting to catch the ball. On examination, he is unable to bend the tip of his right middle finger.

3. A 35-year-old woman is brought into Accident and Emergency acutely short of breath. Her respiratory rate is 50/min. She was involved in a road traffic accident. She has no breath sounds on the left. Her trachea is deviated to the right.

4. An 18-year-old man sustains a stab wound to the right thigh. On examination, he has a large haematoma over the thigh and weak distal pulses. He is unable to move his foot and complains of pins and needles in his foot.

5. A 30-year-old woman involved in a head-on car collision presents with diffuse abdominal pain. Upright chest X-ray shows elevation of the diaphragm with a stomach gas bubble in the left lower lung field.

Question 142
Theme: Diagnosis of fractures and dislocations

Options:

A	Calcaneal fracture	I	March fracture
B	Colles' fracture	J	Galeazzi fracture
C	Anterior shoulder dislocation	K	Greenstick fracture
D	Posterior shoulder dislocation	L	Spiral fracture of the tibia
E	Navicular fracture		
F	Humeral shaft fracture	M	Fracture of the proximal fibula
G	Supracondylar fracture of the humerus		
H	Monteggia's fracture		

For each patient below, choose the SINGLE most likely diagnosis from the above list of options. Each option may be used once, more than once, or not at all.

1. A 33-year-old man, with a history of epilepsy, presents to Casualty following a fit now unable to move his right arm and shoulder. He supports the arm in internal rotation with the other hand.

2. A 26-year-old woman sustains a twisting injury to her left leg while skiing. She has mid-calf swelling and tenderness and is unable to weight-bear.

3. A 10-year-old girl falls and sustains an injury to her right arm. The forearm is stiff, and the hand is deformed. She is only able to extend her fingers when her wrist is passively flexed.

4. A 28-year-old marathon runner complains of pain in the second toe. He ran his last marathon a week ago.

5. A 16-year-old girl falls onto her outstretched hands. She complains of pain and decreased mobility of her right wrist. On examination, she is tender in the anatomical snuffbox.

Question 143
Theme: Diagnosis of gastrointestinal conditions

Options:

A Hepatoma	J Pancreatic pseudocyst
B Oesophageal varices	K Divarication of the recti
C Mallory–Weiss tear	L Acute pancreatitis
D Perforated peptic ulcer	
E Fractured rib	
F Haematoma of the rectus sheath	
G Umbilical hernia	
H Sigmoid volvulus	
I Splenic rupture	

For each case below, choose the SINGLE most likely diagnosis from the above list of options. Each option may be used once, more than once, or not at all.

1. A 50-year-old alcoholic man presents with nausea, vomiting, and epigastric pain. On examination, he has a palpable epigastric mass and a raised amylase. CT scan of the abdomen shows a round well-circumscribed mass in the epigastrium.

2. A 40-year-old multiparous woman presents with a midline abdominal mass. The mass is nontender and appears when she is straining. On examination, the midline mass is visible when she raises her head off the examining bed.

3. A 19-year-old man presents with sudden severe upper abdominal pain after being tackled during rugby practice. He was recently diagnosed with glandular fever.

4. A 7-year-old girl presents with spontaneous massive haematemesis.

5. A 55-year-old male alcoholic presents with vomiting 800 ml of blood. His blood pressure is 80/50 with a pulse rate of 120. He also has ascites.

Question 144
Theme: Causes of cerebral lesions

Options:

A	Arteriovenous malformation	I	Craniopharyngioma
B	Berry aneurysm	J	Meningioma
C	Brain abscess	K	Arteriovenous
D	Extradural haematoma		malformation
E	Subdural haematoma	L	Metastatic carcinoma
F	Carotid artery occlusion		
G	Pituitary adenoma		
H	Medulloblastoma		

For each case below, choose the SINGLE most likely cause from the above list of options. Each option may be used once, more than once, or not at all.

1. A 60-year-old woman treated with total thyroidectomy for thyroid carcinoma now presents with visual changes. On examination, she has bitemporal hemianopsia. CT scan of the head shows a cystic lesion compressing the optic tracts.

2. A 25-year-old man complains of the worst headache of his life. He denies any history of head trauma. He has no focal neurological deficits.

3. A 65-year-old male alcoholic has fluctuating levels of consciousness. He develops focal neurological deficits. His wife reports that he fell down the staircase 2 months ago.

4. A 45-year-old motorcyclist is involved in a road traffic accident. On examination, he has a dilated left pupil and is unconscious. Skull films show a left temporal-parietal fracture.

5. A 55-year-old woman, treated with modified radical mastectomy for breast carcinoma 5 years ago, now presents with gradual onset of confusion and visual disturbances. CT scan of the head shows a cerebral mass.

Question 145
Theme: Causes of dyspnoea

Options:

A Anaemia	J Exacerbation of chronic bronchitis
B Valvular disease	
C Bronchial asthma	K Metastatic carcinoma
D Atelectasis	
E Atypical pneumonia	
F Bronchial carcinoma	
G Acute pulmonary oedema	
H Pulmonary embolus	

For each patient below, choose the SINGLE most likely diagnosis from the above list of options. Each option may be used once, more than once, or not at all.

1. A 33-year-old airline steward presents with a 1-week history of fever, dry cough, and shortness of breath. On examination, he is tachypnoeic. His lungs are clear to auscultation.

2. A 65-year-old man with a history of chronic productive cough now presents to Accident and Emergency short of breath and drowsy.

3. A 60-year-old woman presents with dyspnoea. On examination, she has a firm mass in the left breast and decreased breath sounds in the right lower lung fields. Chest X-ray reveals a pleural effusion.

4. A 50-year-old male patient on the ward awakes with dyspnoea and frothy sputum. He had suffered an MI a week earlier. On examination, he is cyanosed and tachypnoeic. Auscultation of the lung reveals creps.

5. A 40-year-old man presents with cough and breathlessness. Chest X-ray demonstrates diffuse consolidation of the right lower lobe. Despite treatment with intravenous augmentin, the fever persists. Chest X-ray show expansion.

Question 146
Theme: Diagnosis of urological conditions

Options:

A	Carcinoma of the bladder	I	Acute tubular necrosis
B	Carcinoma of the kidney	J	Chronic renal failure
C	Carcinoma of the prostate	K	Ureteric colic
D	Acute pyelonephritis	L	Hydrocoele
E	Testicular torsion		
F	Acute epididymo-orchitis		
G	Testicular tumour		
H	Inflamed Hydatid de Morgani		

For each patient below, choose the SINGLE most likely diagnosis from the above list of options. Each option may be used once, more than once, or not at all.

1. A 26-year-old man presents with a painless lump in his left testis of 6 weeks duration. On examination, he has no inguinal lymphadenopathy. He has an elevated serum alpha-fetoprotein.

2. A 6-year-old boy presents with painless haematuria and scrotal oedema of 2 days duration. His urine demonstrates granular casts.

3. A 70-year-old man presents with poor stream and nocturia. On examination, he has a lemon tinge to his skin, ascites, a palpable bladder and an enlarged prostate gland. His blood pressure is 170/95.

4. A 75-year-old man presents with increased micturition and backache. On examination, he has a palpable bladder and an enlarged prostate. His serum acid phosphatase and alkaline phosphatase are both elevated.

5. A 12-year-old boy presents to Casualty with a red, painful, swollen scrotum. His mid-stream urine is normal.

Question 147
Theme: Diagnosis of cardiovascular diseases in children

Options:

A	Kawasaki disease	J	Toxic synovitis
B	Hereditary angioedema	K	Aortic stenosis
C	Congenital nephrotic syndrome	L	Systemic lupus erythematosus
D	Myocarditis		
E	Pericarditis	M	Paroxysmal atrial tachycardia
F	Primary pulmonary hypertension	N	Mitral stenosis
G	Juvenile rheumatoid arthritis		
H	Acute rheumatic fever		
I	Congestive heart failure		

For each patient below, choose the SINGLE most likely diagnosis from the above list of options. Each option may be used once, more than once, or not at all.

1. A 10-year-old boy presents with stridor. He has a history of recurrent swelling of the hands and feet with abdominal pain and diarrhoea. His sister also suffers from similar attacks.

2. A 6-year-old girl presents with spiking fevers. On examination, she has spindle-shaped swellings of the finger-joints.

3. A 12-year-old boy presents with polyarthritis and abdominal pain. He had a sore throat a week ago. On examination, he is noted to have an early blowing diastolic murmur at the left sternal edge.

4. A 10-year-old boy presents to Casualty following a seizure during gym. On examination, he has a loud systolic ejection murmur with a thrill.

5. A 12-year-old girl presents with pallor, dyspnoea, and a pulse rate of 190. She is noted to have cardiomegaly and hepatomegaly.

Question 148
Theme: The management of obstetric conditions

Options:

A Elective caesarian section
B Epidural anaesthesia
C Ventouse extraction
D Rupture membranes
E Bedrest and control blood
   pressure
F Crash Caesarian section
G IV syntocinon
H Allow vaginal delivery

I Episiotomy

For each case below, choose the SINGLE most appropriate management from the above list of options. Each option may be used once, more than once, or not at all.

1. A 30-year-old female, gravida 2 para 1 with one previous Caesarian section for fetal distress, presents at 38 weeks with regular uterine contractions and with the fetal head engaged.

2. A 20-year-old primiparous woman presents with uterine contractions for the past 14 hours. On examination, the os is 6 cm dilated. The membranes are intact. The fetal heart rate is 140/min.

3. A 21-year-old multiparous woman presents with uterine contractions for the past 18 hours. On examination, the os is 9 cm dilated and the presenting part is at the level of the ischial spines. The fetal heart monitor shows a variable deceleration with a fetal heart rate of 100/min.

4. A 20-year-old primigravida of 36 weeks gestation presents with a blood pressure of 160/110.

5. A 35-year-old second para is admitted in labour. However she suddenly ruptures her membranes with drainage of meconium stained liquor and prolapse of the umbilical cord. The fetal heart monitor shows a fetal heart rate of 100/min.

Question 149
Theme: The treatment of gynaecological conditions

Options:

A	Laparoscopy	I	Hysterectomy alone
B	Colposcopy	J	Excision with diathermy
C	Suction curettage	K	5-fluorouracil cream
D	Post-coital pill	L	Myomectomy
E	Intravenous antibiotics	M	Cone biopsy
F	Total abdominal hysterectomy and bilateral salpingo-oophorectomy		
G	Urgent resuscitation and laparotomy		
H	Papanicolou smear		

For each presentation below, choose the SINGLE most appropriate treatment from the above list of options. Each option may be used once, more than once, or not at all.

1. A 28-year-old woman is noted to have an abnormal cervical smear that demonstrates condyloma accuminata.

2. A 20-year-old woman presents to the casualty with severe right-sided abdominal pain and left shoulder pain. She stopped taking the pill 2 months ago and has not menstruated since. Her blood pressure is 90/50 mmHg and her pulse rate is 120/min.

3. An 18-year-old primigravida of 12 weeks gestation would like to terminate her pregnancy.

4. A 30-year-old nulliparous woman complains of infertility. She has regular periods that are heavy and last for 8 days. She and her husband have been trying to conceive for over a year now. Her husband has seen a urologist and been cleared, and she wonders if she is at fault. Her ovulation test is normal. Ultrasound reveals uterine fibroids.

5. A 70-year-old woman presents with a 3-month history of vaginal bleeding. Pipelle endometrial sampling and curettage reveal adenocarcinoma.

Question 150
Theme: Diagnosis of psychiatric conditions

Options:

A	Pica	J	Fugue
B	Formication	K	Cocaine intoxication
C	Alcohol withdrawal	L	Opioid withdrawal
D	Alcohol intoxication	M	Drug toxicity
E	Schizophrenia		
F	Xenophobia		
G	Agoraphobia		
H	Algophobia		
I	Delirium		

For each patient below, choose the SINGLE most likely diagnosis from the above list of options. Each option may be used once, more than once, or not at all.

1. A 2-year-old boy presents with anaemia and abdominal pain. His mother states that she has seen him peeling paint chips off the wall and wonders if he has been eating this.

2. A 23-year-old woman becomes afraid to leave her home. She functions normally except will not step outside her house.

3. An 18-year-old man presents with nausea, vomiting and diaphoresis. His pupils are dilated, and his blood pressure is elevated. He has a history of drug addiction.

4. A 30-year-old woman is found in an amnestic state. Her husband reports that she had been missing for a few days after she had been served with divorce papers.

5. A 30-year-old man with bipolar disorder is taking lithium. He was recently started on thiazide diuretics for mild hypertension. He is now confused with ataxia, blurred vision, and a coarse tremor.

Question 151
Theme: Causes of infection

Options:

A   *Escherichia coli*
B   *Staphylococcus aureus*
C   Group A streptococcus
D   *Staphylococcus epidermidis*
E   Group B streptococcus
F   *Clostridium perfringens*
G   *Klebsiella pneumoniae*
H   *Proteus mirabilis*
I   *Mycobacterium tuberculosis*

J   *Enterobacter aerogenes*

For each case below, choose the SINGLE most likely organism from the above list of options. Each option may be used once, more than once, or not at all.

1. A 20-year-old woman presents with dysuria. She has no prior history of urinary tract infections. Urinalysis demonstrates white cells and pus.

2. A 30-year-old multiparous woman presents with spiking fever and a foul-smelling vaginal discharge 24 hours after delivery of her baby.

3. A 55-year-old woman presents with back pain. Investigations reveal a pyogenic vertebral osteomyelitis.

4. A 40-year-old woman presents with dysuria and urinary incontinence. Her urine is noted to be alkaline.

5. A 50-year-old diabetic woman presents with fever, redness, swelling, and pain over the right side of her face.

Question 152
Theme: The treatment of infections

Options:

A	Vancomycin	J	Amoxicillin
B	Flucloxacillin	K	Pentamidine
C	Trimethoprim		
D	Gentamicin		
E	Penicillin		
F	Cefotaxime		
G	Erythromycin		
H	Tetracycline		
I	Rifampicin, isoniazid and pyrazinamide		

For each case below, choose the SINGLE most appropriate antibiotic treatment from the above list of options. Each option may be used once, more than once, or not at all.

1. A 4-year-old child presents to Accident and Emergency with high fever and stridorous breathing. He is sitting forward and drooling saliva. He requires intubation for respiratory distress.

2. A 60-year-old man presents with urinary retention on the ward. He had undergone elective abdominal aortic aneurysm repair in the morning. Foley catheterisation is suggested.

3. A 60-year-old woman presents with dysuria and increased frequency of micturition. She has white cells and pus in her urine.

4. A 20-year-old man presents with a neck mass in the posterior triangle. Fine needle aspirate demonstrates acid fast bacilli.

5. A 60-year-old male patient presents with diarrhoea on the ward. He has been on broad-spectrum intravenous antibiotics for several weeks for a discharging fistula post total hip replacement.

Question 153
Theme: Investigations of paediatric emergencies

Options:

A   Full blood count (FBC)
B   Serum glucose
C   Skull X-ray
D   Chest X-ray
E   Urinanalysis
F   ESR
G   Serum urea and electrolytes
H   Computed tomography scan of the head
I   Lateral soft-tissue neck X-ray

For each case below, choose the SINGLE most discriminating investigation from the above list of options. Each option may be used once, more than once, or not at all.

1. An 8-month-old baby is brought to casualty by her mother after falling off the sofa on to her head. On examination, she is irritable and alert with no lateralising signs. There is a haematoma over her left occiput.

2. A 6-year-old girl is brought to casualty by her mother after falling off a climbing frame in the school playground. On examination, she has no deformity or swelling of her extremities. Instead she has bruising of various colours over her arms and she has tender ribs to palpation.

3. A 2-year-old girl is brought to casualty by her father after falling down the stairs. She is drowsy and has vomited twice. On examination, she has a swelling over her occiput. Her pupils are sluggish to respond. Her blood pressure is 120/70, and her pulse rate is 60.

4. A 2-year-old boy has swallowed a 50 pence coin and points to his throat. He is not distressed.

5. A 16-year-old girl presents to casualty with an uncontrollable spontaneous nose bleed. She has bruising of various ages over her extremities.

Options:

A Middle cerebral artery infarction
B Spinal artery occlusion
C Guillain–Barré syndrome
D Polio
E Deep venous thrombosis
F Acute cord compression
G Intermittent claudication
H Critical limb ischaemia
I Compartment syndrome

For each case below, choose the SINGLE most likely cause from the above list of options. Each option may be used once, more than once, or not at all.

1. A 67-year-old male smoker presents with pain in his left calf on walking and also at rest. His ankle-brachial doppler pressure index is 0.3.

2. A 30-year-old man develops gradual weakness in his extremities following the flu. On examination, he is unable to raise his legs and has loss of muscle tone and deep tendon reflexes. The lumbar puncture demonstrates 4 lymphocytes/cc, 2 g/L of protein, and 3 mmol/L of glucose.

3. A 20-year-old man presents with pain on the inner aspect of his right knee after being tackled in rugby. He reports a tearing sensation and is unable to move his leg. On examination, the knee is swollen and tender, and the joint is locked.

4. A 70-year-old woman with a history of multiple myeloma suddenly develops back pain and is unable to move her legs. On examination, she has hypotonia, loss of deep tendon reflexes, and sensory loss of her lower extremities. She also goes into urinary retention.

5. A 2-year-old boy presents with pain in the calves and inability to move his lower legs. He is also noted to have pneumonia and splenomegaly. On examination, he has loss of motor power and tone, loss of sensation, and decreased deep tendon reflexes in his lower extremities.

Question 155
Theme: Principles and practice of evidence-based medicine

Options:

    A   True
    B   False

For each statement below, choose the SINGLE correct response from the above list of options.

1. Evidence-based medicine is cookbook medicine.

2. Evidence-based medicine is restricted to randomised trials and meta-analyses.

3. Evidence-based medicine involves obtaining the best external evidence with which to answer our clinical questions.

4. Evidence-based medicine involves using individual clinical expertise or the best available external evidence to treat a patient.

5. Evidence-based medicine is the conscientious, explicit, and judicious use of the current best evidence in making decisions about the care of individual patients.

6. Evidence-based medicine suggests we determine the accuracy of a diagnostic test by a randomised trial of patients harbouring the relevant disorder.

7. Evidence-based medicine suggests that the standard for judging the efficacy of a treatment should be based on the systematic review of several randomised trials.

8. Evidence-based medicine suggests we accept the next best external evidence if no randomised trial has been carried out for a particular patient's predicament.

9. Evidence-based medicine is an attempt to lower the cost of patient's care.

10. Evidence-based medicine can be conducted from the armchair.

Question 156
Theme: Diagnosis of obstetric conditions

Options:

A	Mittelschmerz		J	Eclampsia
B	Ectopic pregnancy		K	Endometritis
C	Abruptio placentae		L	Endometriosis
D	Postpartum haemorrhage			
E	Early pregnancy			
F	Quickening			
G	Braxton-Hicks contractions			
H	Placenta praevia			
I	Pregnancy induced hypertension			

For each case below, choose the SINGLE most likely diagnosis from the above list of options. Each option may be used once, more than once, or not at all.

1. A 30-year-old multiparous woman presents with scant vaginal bleeding, severe hypotension and a tender uterus. Fetal heart sounds are not detected.

2. A 26-year-old multiparous woman presents with painless irregular contractions in her third trimester of pregnancy.

3. A 20-year-old primigravid woman is brought into casualty following a fit in her 36th week of pregnancy. She is noted to have a blood pressure of 170/110 and 2+ proteinuria.

4. A 22-year-old primigravid woman is seen in clinic at 28 weeks. She is noted to have ankle oedema and a blood pressure of 160/110. Her urine demonstrates the presence of protein.

5. A 28-year-old primigravid woman presents with lower abdominal pain and a spiking fever 24 hours after delivery of her baby.

Question 157
Theme: The management of postoperative complications

Options:

A	Intravenous calcium gluconate	I	Mid-stream urine for culture
B	Insulin in dextrose	J	Intravenous hydro-cortisone
C	Potassium replacement		
D	Intravenous saline and frusemide		
E	Check serum urea and creatinine		
F	Check full blood count		
G	Obtain KUB film		
H	Obtain chest X-ray		

For each case below, choose the SINGLE most appropriate management from the above list of options. Each option may be used once, more than once, or not at all.

1. A 40-year-old woman started on gentamicin in the recovery room suddenly stops breathing. She had received a neuro-muscular blocking agent in surgery.

2. A 50-year-old man develops postoperative hypotension and oliguria following bowel surgery. An ECG shows prolonged PR interval and QRS interval, loss of P waves, and depression of the ST segment.

3. A 70-year-old man develops tinnitus and deafness after surgery. His medications include gentamicin and frusemide.

4. A 40-year-old woman has undergone intestinal bypass surgery for gross obesity. She now presents with pain in the lumbar region and haematuria. She is apyrexial.

5. A 40-year-old woman with systemic lupus erythematosus develops nausea, vomiting and severe abdominal pain follow-ing cholecystectomy. She becomes hypotensive and tachy-cardic. She is noted to have an irregular tan and denies sun-exposure.

Question 158
Theme: The management of postoperative complications

Options:

A	Intravenous dantrolene sodium	J	Obtain abdominal X-ray
B	Intravenous calcium gluconate	K	Check full blood count
C	Blood transfusion		
D	Blood cultures		
E	Obtain chest X-ray		
F	Mid-stream urine collection for culture		
G	Intravenous broad-spectrum antibiotics		
H	Insulin in dextrose		
I	Foley catheterisation		

For each case below, choose the SINGLE most appropriate management option from the above list of options. Each option may be used once, more than once, or not at all.

1. A 30-year-old female post appendicectomy develops high fever of 42°C, hypotension, and mottled cyanosis in the recovery room. She received halothane inhalation gas in surgery. She was noted to have trismus during intubation.

2. A 40-year-old man complains of circumoral numbness following thyroidectomy. Tapping over his preauricular regon elicits facial twitching.

3. A 50-year-old man post nephrectomy becomes febrile, confused, tachypnoeic, and tachycardic. He was recently advanced to a soft diet. He has no bowel sounds.

4. A 60-year-old man post cholecystectomy complains of lower abdominal pain. On examination, his bladder is palpable at the umbilicus.

5. A 70-year-old woman post total hip replacement becomes tachypnoeic. She is pale and hypotensive.

Question 159
Theme: Causes of neurological signs

Options:

A   Middle cerebral artery infarction
B   Anterior cerebral artery infarction
C   Posterior cerebral artery infarction
D   Vertebrobasilar ischaemia
E   Subacute combined degeneration of the cord
F   Syringomyelia
G   Cord compression
H   Tabes dorsalis

For each case below, choose the SINGLE most likely cause from the above list of options. Each option may be used once, more than once, or not at all.

1. A 50-year-old man presents with severe stabbing pains in his chest and limbs. He walks with a wide-based gait. On examination, he has ptosis and small, irregular pupils that react to accommodation but not to light. He has absent deep tendon reflexes and position sense.

2. A 60-year-old man presents with urinary incontinence and contralateral paresis of the foot, leg and shoulder. He is awake but silent and immobile, in a coma-vigil state.

3. A 70-year-old man presents with contralateral hemisensory loss and paresis of conjugate gaze to the opposite side.

4. A 70-year-old man presents with dysarthria and incontractable hiccups. On examination, he has nystagmus and is noted to have an ataxic gait.

5. A 40-year-old alcoholic man presents with numbness and tingling sensation in his feet. He is noted to have loss of vibration and position senses in his legs with loss of deep tendon reflexes. Full blood count reveals a macrocytic anaemia.

Question 160
Theme: Causes of ascites

Options:

A   Tuberculous peritonitis
B   Meig's syndrome
C   Budd–Chiari syndrome
D   Constrictive pericarditis
E   Portal vein thrombosis
F   Compression of the portal vein by lymph nodes
G   Cirrhosis
H   Right heart failure due to mitral stenosis
I   Pseudomyxoma peritonei
J   Protein-losing enteropathies

For each case below, choose the SINGLE most likely cause from the above list of options. Each option may be used once, more than once, or not at all.

1. A 40-year-old woman presents with ovarian fibroma, right hydrothorax and ascites.

2. A 25-year-old woman develops nausea, vomiting, and abdominal pain. On examination, she has tender hepatomegaly and ascites. She was recently started on oral contraceptives.

3. A 30-year-old man develops ascites and right lower quadrant colicky pain. The ascitic fluid is viscous and mucinoid in nature.

4. A 40-year-old woman presents with ascites. On examination, she has a dominant 'a' wave in the JVP, a loud pulmonary second sound and a low volume peripheral artery pulse volume. She has a history of rheumatic fever.

5. A 50-year-old woman presents with fatigue and ascites. She is noted to have a rapid, irregular pulse rate with small volume. The chest X-ray reveals a small heart with calcification seen on the lateral view. The 12-lead ECG demonstrates low QRS voltage and T wave inversion.

Question 161
Theme: Causes of poisoning

Options:

A	Lead	J	Paraquat
B	Paracetamol	K	Ethylene glycol
C	Salicylate	L	Methanol
D	Arsenic		
E	Ethanol		
F	Mercury		
G	Cyanide		
H	Carbon monoxide		
I	Organophosphate insecticides		

For each case below, choose the SINGLE most likely cause from the above list of options. Each option may be used once, more than once, or not at all.

1. A 4-year-old child presents with anorexia, nausea and vomiting. On examination, he has a blue line on the gums and is noted to have a foot drop. Blood test reveals anaemia.

2. A 16-year-old girl presents with weakness, excessive salivation, vomiting, abdominal pain and diarrhoea. There is 'raindrop' pigmentation of the skin. Diagnosis is made from nail clippings.

3. A 40-year-old farmer presents with acute shortness of breath and headache. His skin is red in colour, and he smells of bitter almonds.

4. A 40-year-old woman complains of headache and memory impairment following the installation of a gas fireplace. Her skin colour is pink.

5. A 50-year-old agricultural farmer presents with nausea, vomiting, hypersalivation, and bronchospasm.

Question 162
Theme: Diagnosis of psychiatric disorders

Options:

A	Munchausen's syndrome	I	Parkinson's disease
B	Alcohol withdrawal delirium	J	Cushing's syndrome
C	Extrapyramidal side-effect	K	Autonomic side-effect of
D	Hypothyroidism		drug
E	Hysterical neurosis	L	Anticholinergic side-
F	Acromegaly		effect of drug
G	Dissociative disorder		
H	Malingering disorder		

For each patient below, choose the SINGLE most likely diagnosis from the above list of options. Each option may be used once, more than once, or not at all.

1. A 28-year-old female presents with lower abdominal pain. On examination, she has multiple surgical scars over her abdomen. Her abdominal and pelvic examinations are normal. She insists she needs a laparoscopy.

2. A 50-year-old schizophrenic is started on haloperidol. A month later he is noted to be drooling saliva and walking with a shuffling gait. He also suffers from involuntary chewing movements.

3. A 40-year-old female complains of dry mouth, blurry vision, and constipation. On examination, she has dilated pupils. She was started on amitryptiline for major depression.

4. A 45-year-old man complains of headaches, excessive thirst, and frequent urination. On examination, he is noted to have bad acne, coarse skin and has a goitre. He has moved his wedding band to the 5th finger.

5. A 30-year-old man presents to casualty with a dislocated shoulder. On examination, the shoulder is found not to be dislocated. The patient insists it is dislocated.

Question 163
Theme: Diagnosis of conditions which mimic physical disease

Options:

A   Conversion disorder
B   Histrionic personality disorder
C   Body dysmorphic disorder
D   Briquet's syndrome
E   Munchausen syndrome
F   Hypochondriacal neurosis
G   Somatoform pain disorder

For each patient below, choose the SINGLE most likely diagnosis from the above list of options. Each option may be used once, more than once, or not at all.

1. A 40-year-old man insists that his leg is gangrenous and needs to be amputated. On examination, he has normal extremities.

2. A 30-year-old woman presents with a history of multiorgan ailments. She reports that she has always been poorly ever since she was a child. She sees her GP on a regular basis and each time for a different medical symptom. No medical abnormalities can be found. She has multiple surgical scars over her entire body.

3. A 50-year-old man facing redundancy is now paralysed in both legs and wheelchair-bound. The paralysis and sensory loss is inconsistent with the anatomical distribution of nerves.

4. A 40-year-old woman after failing her driver's test complains of chest pain. No medical cause can be identified.

5. A 50-year-old man insists he has throat cancer. He has shopped around and can find no doctor who will concur with him. He visits his GP frequently.

Question 164
Theme: Principles and practice of clinical governance

Options:
    A   True
    B   False

For each statement below, choose the SINGLE correct response from the above list of options.

1. Clinical governance is the means by which organisations ensure the provision of quality clinical care by making individuals accountable for setting, maintaining and monitoring performance standards.

2. Clinical governance comprises corporate accountability for clinical performance, internal and external mechanisms for improving clinical performance.

3. NHS trust chief executives are financially accountable.

4. NHS trust chief executives are accountable for the performance of its practitioners and the quality of care they deliver.

5. Health professionals may set their own standards of professional practice, conduct and discipline.

6. The Commission for Health Improvement will support, reinforce and facilitate clinical governance in all NHS Trusts.

7. The National Institute for Clinical Excellence will develop information about improving standards of access and treatment country-wide.

8. Clinical governance emphasises lifelong learning and professional development.

9. Clinical governance discourages individual practitioners to voice concerns if differences in practice are observed.

10. Clinical governance discourages evidence-based practice.

Question 165
Theme: Diagnosis of genetic disorders and birth defects

Options:

A	Down's syndrome	J	Trisomy 18
B	Turner's syndrome	J	Prader–Willi syndrome
C	Klinefelter's syndrome	K	Fragile X syndrome
D	Alport's syndrome		
E	Trisomy 13		
F	Waardenburg's syndrome		
G	Treacher–Collins syndrome		
H	Marfan's syndrome		
I	Fanconi's syndrome		

For each case below, choose the SINGLE most likely diagnosis from the above list of options. Each option may be used once, more than once, or not at all.

1. A newborn is noted to have microcephaly, cleft lip, and palate and polydactyly.

2. A child is noted to have a white forelock, wide-set eyes, and a sensorineural hearing loss.

3. A baby is noted to have eye signs of prominent epicanthal folds and tiny pale spots on the iris forming a ring around the pupil. He has a single transverse palmar crease and a short, incurved little finger. There is a wide gap between the first and second toes. His limbs are hypotonic and hyperextensible.

4. A newborn girl is noted to have lymphoedema of the hands and feet and a systolic heart murmur.

5. A 4-year-old boy presents with central obesity. He has almond-shaped palpebral fissures and a down-turned mouth. He has small genitalia.

Question 166
Theme: Specific tests for infectious diseases

Options:

A   Paul Bunnell
B   VDRL
C   Ziehl–Neelsen stain for AFB
D   ASO
E   Widal
F   Weil-Felix
G   ELISA
H   Gram stain
I   Schuffner agglutination test

For each case below, choose the SINGLE most specific test from the above list of options. Each option may be used once, more than once, or not at all.

1. A 25-year-old man presents unwell with a 2-day history of fever, headache, and vomiting. He is noted to have an eschar. You suspect typhus.

2. A 30-year-old man presents with fever, headache, and diarrhoea. He is noted to have rose spots on his trunk.

3. A 23-year-old man presents with a red maculopapular rash on his soles and anal papules.

4. A 30-year-old man presents with fever, jaundice, and painful calves. He is an avid swimmer. You suspect Weil's disease.

5. A 20-year-old female presents with sore throat and is noted to have petechiae on the palate.

Question 167
Theme: Diagnosis of chest injuries

Options:

A	Flail chest	H	Diaphragmatic rupture
B	Tension pneumothorax	I	Open pneumothorax
C	Haemothorax		
D	Cardiac tamponade		
E	Rib fracture		
F	Pulmonary contusion		
G	Myocardial contusion		

For each case below, choose the SINGLE most likely diagnosis from the above list of options. Each option may be used once, more than once, or not at all.

1. A 50-year-old man sustains blunt trauma to his chest and presents with marked dyspnoea. A nasogastric tube is inserted to decompress his stomach. On chest X-ray, the nasogastric tube is seen in the left side of the chest.

2. A 55-year-old man involved in a road traffic accident complains of chest pain. He was driving the car and rear-ended the front car with some force. A friction rub is elicited. His ECG shows multiple premature ventricular ectopic beats.

3. A 30-year-old man is stabbed in the back and is brought to Accident and Emergency in respiratory distress. His blood pressure is 90/50 with a pulse rate of 110. He has dull breath sounds over his left chest. You leave the knife in situ.

4. A 40-year-old man is stabbed in the chest and is brought to Accident and Emergency with shortness of breath. A 4 cm stab wound is noted, and the wound is heard to 'suck' with each breath.

5. A 30-year-old man is stabbed in the left side of his chest and is brought to Accident and Emergency. He is short of breath and restless. His chest is clear to auscultation. There is a rise in venous pressure with inspiration. The chest X-ray shows a globular-shaped heart.

Question 168
Theme: The management of head injuries

Options:

A Admit for neurological observation

B Assess adequacy of breathing

C Removal of penetrating object

D Discharge with head injury advice

E Detailed neurological assessment

F Airway assessment with cervical spine control

G Assess circulation and maintain adequate perfusion

H Neurosurgical consultation

I Obtain urgent CT scan of the head

J Intubate the patient

K Pronounce the patient as deceased

For each case below, choose the SINGLE most appropriate form of management from the above list of options. Each option may be used once, more than once, or not at all.

1. A 30-year-old cyclist is struck by a car in a head-on collision and arrives intubated to Accident and Emergency. Upon arrival, his Glasgow Coma Scale is 3. He has fixed and dilated pupils.

2. A 60-year-old man is brought to Accident and Emergency following assault and battery to the head. He has a face mask and reservoir bag delivering 15 L/min of oxygen, a stiff cervical collar and is attached to an intravenous drip. He has no spontaneous eye opening except to pain, makes incomprehensible sounds, and does not obey commands. He demonstrates flexion withdrawal to painful stimuli. On suction, he has no gag reflex.

3. A 20-year-old man involved in an RTA presents to Accident and Emergency with a large open scalp wound, multiple facial injuries and a deformed right tibia.

4. A 40-year-old man is brought to Casualty with a knife impaled in his occiput.

5. A 30-year-old female involved in an RTA with multiple injuries is brought to Casualty intubated with adequate oxygen delivery. Her blood pressure is noted to be 80/50 with a pulse of 120.

Question 169
Theme: The management of back pain

Options:

A   Obtain chest X-ray   I   Abdominal ultrasound
B   Bedrest for 2 weeks
C   Rest for 2 days with analgesia
D   Physiotherapy
E   Urinanalysis
F   Investigate for underlying
    tumour or other bone
    pathology
G   Urgent orthopaedic referral
    for surgical decompression
H   Routine orthopaedic referral
    for decompression of nerve root

For each case below, choose the SINGLE most appropriate management option from the above list of options. Each option may be used once, more than once, or not at all.

1. A 40-year-old man complains of lower back pain after moving heavy furniture. He has no associated nerve root findings.

2. A 50-year-old female complain of back pain worse at night. X-ray of her spine shows crush fractures of two vertebrae. She denies trauma.

3. A 60-year-old man presents with back pain radiating bilaterally below the knees. On examination, he has saddle anaesthesia, urinary incontinence and loss of anal tone.

4. A 50-year-old female complains of chronic lower back pain radiating into her buttocks. There is no evidence of nerve root entrapment.

5. A 30-year-old man complains of back pain radiating below the knee. On examination, he has sensory loss over the lateral aspect of the right calf and medial aspect of the right foot. He is unable to dorsiflex his great toe. He has tried bedrest for 6 weeks!

Question 170
Theme: The treatment of fractures

Options:

A   Collar and cuff sling
B   Broad arm sling
C   Open reduction and internal fixation
D   Closed reduction and plaster immobilisation
E   Hemiarthroplasty
F   Skeletal traction
G   Skin traction
H   External fixation
I   Gallows traction

For each case below, choose the SINGLE most appropriate treatment from the above list of options. Each option may be used once, more than once, or not at all.

1. A 12-year-old boy is injured in rugby. He sustained a blow to his chest. He complains of pain around the shoulder. X-ray reveals a fracture of the middle third of the clavicle with displacement.

2. A 6-year-old girl falls onto the side of her left arm and now complains of left shoulder pain. On examination, she has numbness over the 'regimental badge' area. X-ray reveals a greenstick fracture of the proxial humerus.

3. A 55-year-old woman presents with pain in her upper arm without a history of trauma. Examination reveals intact radial nerve and brachial artery. X-ray demonstrates a transverse fracture of the humerus with a lytic lesion at the fracture site.

4. A 60-year-old woman with a history of breast carcinoma presents with pain in her right thigh. X-ray reveals a transverse fracture of the femur.

5. An 18-month-old baby is brought to Casualty after a fall unable to weight-bear. X-ray reveals a spiral fracture of the femur.

Question 171
Theme: Diagnosis of head injuries

Options:

A	Basal skull fracture	H	Extradural haematoma
B	Depressed skull fracture	I	Open skull fracture
C	Compound skull fracture	J	Brain contusion
D	Diffuse axonal injury		
E	Concussion		
F	Subdural haematoma		
G	Intracerebral haemorrhage		

For each case below, choose the SINGLE most likely diagnosis from the above list of options. Each option may be used once, more than once, or not at all.

1. A 30-year-old female involved in an RTA is brought by ambulance to Accident and Emergency. She is noted to have bruising of the mastoid process and periorbital haematoma. On otoscopic examination, she has bleeding behind the tympanic membrane.

2. A 60-year-old man was kicked in the head a week ago. He is brought to Accident and Emergency in an unconscious state. He smells of alcohol. On examination, he has a rising BP and unequal pupils. His GCS is 8.

3. A 40-year-old man was struck in the head by a cricket ball. He had an episode of loss of consciousness lasting 5 minutes. The patient now complains of headache. He has no lateralising signs on neurological examination.

4. A 50-year-old man with a history of epilepsy has a fit and strikes the side of his head on the edge of the bathtub. He is dazed and complains of headache. Skull X-ray reveals a linear fracture of the parietal area. His level of consciousness diminishes.

5. A 60-year-old man is struck in the head with a dustbin lid and presents with an open scalp wound. Skull X-ray confirms an underlying skull fracture. The dura is intact.

Question 172
Theme: The treatment of shoulder region injuries

Options:

A	Broad arm sling	G	Hippocratic technique
B	Collar and cuff sling	H	Kocher's technique
C	Rest and analgaesia then mobilise	I	Surgical repair
D	Injection of local anaesthetic and steroids		
E	Manipulation under anaesthesia		
F	Traction on the arm in 90 degrees of abduction and externally rotate the arm		

For each case below, choose the SINGLE most appropriate treatment from the above list of options. Each option may be used once, more than once, or not at all.

1. A 20-year-old man presents with shoulder pain and decreased range of movement after being struck in the upper back. X-ray reveals fracture of the scapula.

2. A 60-year-old builder presents with pain in the upper arm. On examination, he has a low bulge of the muscle belly of the long head of biceps.

3. A 50-year-old man complains of pain in his shoulder. The pain is elicited in abduction between an arc of 60 and 120 degrees. He reports that he has always had shoulder trouble.

4. A 20-year-old rugby player falls onto the point of his shoulder and complains of shoulder tip pain. The lateral end of the clavicle is very prominent.

5. A 30-year-old hiker falls onto his outstretched hand and injures his right shoulder. On examination, there is loss of the rounded shoulder contour with prominence of the acromion. On palpation, there is a gap beneath the acromion, and the humeral head is palpable in the axilla. The nearest hospital is 6 hours hike away, and you are alone with him up on the mountain. You cannot obtain a signal on your mobile phone. You decide to treat the patient.

Question 173
Theme: Causes of painful knee

Options:

A	Reiter's syndrome	I	Rheumatoid arthritis
B	Meniscal tear	J	Posterior cruciate ligament rupture
C	Rupture of the patellar tendon		
D	Osgood-Schlatter's syndrome	K	Anterior cruciate ligament rupture
E	Septic arthritis		
F	Ankylosing spondylitis	L	Collateral ligament injury
G	Osteoarthritis	M	Tumour of the bone and cartilage
H	Gout		
		N	Osteomyelitis

For each case below, choose the SINGLE most likely cause from the above list of options. Each option may be used once, more than once, or not at all.

1. A 20-year-old female presents with a painful locked knee following a twisting injury. There is no immediate haemarthrosis.

2. A 30-year-old female passenger strikes her shin against the car dashboard in an RTA and now complains of severe knee pain. On examination, she has profound haemarthrosis. The knee is immobilised in plaster to prevent flexion.

3. A 30-year-old female twists her knee while skiing and now presents with an acutely painful swollen knee. Aspiration of the haemarthrosis eases the pain and you are able to examine the knee. With the knee flexed at 90 degrees, you are able to pull the tibia forwards on the femur by 1 cm.

4. A 10-year-old boy on prednisolone presents with a painful swollen knee. He recently had a chest infection. He is now unable to move the knee at all. There is a joint effusion present.

5. A 50-year-old woman presents with myalgia, fever and a painful swollen knee. She denies trauma. She has a raised ESR and CRP. X-ray shows some bony erosion.

Question 174
Theme: The treatment of diabetic complications

Options:

A   Insulin sliding scale, heparin and 0.9% normal saline
B   Insulin sliding scale, heparin and 0.45% normal saline
C   Insulin sliding scale, 0.9% normal saline and potassium replacement
D   Insulin sliding scale, 0.45% normal saline and potassium replacement
E   50 ml of 50% dextrose IV
F   Sugary drink
G   Chest X-ray
H   Measure C-peptide levels

For each case below, choose the SINGLE most appropriate treatment from the above list of options. Each option may be used once, more than once, or not at all.

1. A 67-year-old man is noted to have a glucose of 37 mmol/L and a Na of 163 mmol/L. He has no prior history of diabetes and has been on intravenous fluids for a week. His other medications include IV cefuroxime, metronidazole, and dexamethasone.

2. A 60-year-old man is brought into Accident and Emergency in an unconscious state. His glucose is 35 mmol/L. His arterial blood gas shows a pH 7.2 and a paCO$_2$ of 2. Serum Na is 140, K is 3.0, Cl is 100, and the HCO$_3$ is 5 mmol/L.

3. A 40-year-old diabetic actor is started on propranolol for stage-fright. He collapses after a day shooting. He has not changed his insulin regime. His glucose is 1.5 mmol/L.

4. A 50-year-old diabetic presents in a coma. He is febrile with diminished breath sounds on auscultation. He has warm extremities. His glucose is 20 mmol. His white count is 22 with increased neutrophils.

5. A 50-year-old woman presents with tachycardia, sweating and agitation. Her husband is a diabetic. She has a history of Munchausen's syndrome.

Question 175
Theme: Diagnosis of hand injuries

Options:

A Mallet finger
B Bennett's fracture
C Median nerve injury
D Radial nerve injury
E Ulnar nerve injury
F Boutonniere deformity
G Flexor digitorum profundus injury
H Flexor digitorum superficialis injury
I Ulnar collateral ligament injury

For each case below, choose the SINGLE most likely diagnosis from the above list of options. Each option may be used once, more than once, or not at all.

1. A 40-year-old woman presents with drooping of the terminal phalanx of her middle right finger. She was making the bed at the time of injury. She is now unable to extend the tip of her finger.

2. A 45-year-old man presents with lacerations to the hand from cut glass. You hold all three uninjured fingers in extension and ask him to flex the lacerated finger. He is unable to comply.

3. A 20-year-old man with a history of depression presents with slashed wrists. You ask the patient to place the back of his hand flat on the table and have him point his thumb to the ceiling against resistance. He is unable to comply.

4. A 40-year-old man presents with numbness in his palm after falling and hitting the heel of his hand against the pavement. The distribution of numbness is over the palmar aspect of the 4th and 5th digits.

5. A 30-year-old woman sustains injury to her hand while skiing. She complains of pain around the metacarpophalangeal joint of her thumb and has difficulty abducting her thumb. She has loss of pincer ability.

Question 176
Theme: Causes of a painful foot

Options:

A   Morton's neuroma
B   Stress fracture
C   Avulsion fracture
D   Jones fracture
E   Hallux fracture
F   Plantar fasciitis
G   Osteochondritis – Freiberg's
    disease
H   Metatarsalgia

I   Osteochondritis –
    Kohler's disease
J   Bunion
K   Gout

For each case below, choose the SINGLE most likely cause from the above list of options. Each option may be used once, more than once, or not at all.

1. A 50-year-old man presents with pain over the medial calcaneum and pain on dorsiflexion and eversion of the forefoot.

2. A 60-year-old man complains of continual pain in his forefoot worse when walking. X-ray shows widening and flattening of the second metatarsal head and degenerative changes in the metatarsophalangeal joint.

3. A 50-year-old woman complains of painful shooting pains in her right foot when walking. She is tender in the third/fourth toe interspace.

4. A 30-year-old soldier complains of pain in his foot when weight-bearing. X-ray shows no fracture. He is tender around the proximal fifth metatarsal bone.

5. A 20-year-old man complains of pain over the lateral aspect of his right foot. X-ray shows a transverse fracture of the basal shaft of the 5th metatarsal bone.

Question 177
Theme: The management of neck injuries

Options:

- A Repeat C-spine X-ray
- B Skull traction
- C Cervical collar
- D Surgical decompression and stabilisation
- E Anti-inflammatories and physiotherapy
- F Reduction and immobilisation in a halo-body cast
- G Immobilisation in a halo-body cast

For each case below, choose the SINGLE most appropriate treatment option from the above list of options. Each option may be used once, more than once, or not at all.

1. A 30-year-old female complains of headache and painful stiff neck following a whiplash injury sustained 24 hours ago. She has no neurological findings. X-ray shows loss of the normal lordotic curve of the spine.

2. A 25-year-old female involved in an RTA is found to have an unstable fracture of C1 with disruption of the arch.

3. A 30-year-old man involved in an RTA is sent to X-ray wearing a hard cervical collar with sandbags secured on either side of his head. The cervical X-ray shows no abnormalities of all 7 vertebrae down to the C6/C7 junction. He has no neck pain. He has no focal neurological signs.

4. A 19-year-old man involved in a high-velocity RTA is found to have a displaced fracture of the odontoid peg.

5. A 25-year-old female sustains head injuries going through the windshield of her car in a high-speed RTA. X-ray shows undisplaced fracture of the pedicle of C2.

Question 178
Theme: Diagnosis of cardiovascular diseases

Options:

A	Angina pectoralis	I	Mitral regurgitation
B	Aortic stenosis	J	Congestive cardio-
C	Tricuspid regurgitation		myopathy
D	Aortic regurgitation	K	Mitral stenosis
E	Myocardial infarction	L	Restrictive cardio-
F	Acute pericarditis		myopathy
G	Hypertrophic obstructive	M	Constrictive pericarditis
	cardiomyopathy	N	Dressler's syndrome

For each case below, choose the SINGLE most likely diagnosis from the above list of options. Each option may be used once, more than once, or not at all.

1. A 40-year-old man presents with inspiratory chest pain two months after a heart attack. On examination, a friction rub is heard in both systole and diastole. The ECG shows ST elevation throughout.

2. A 35-year-old IVDA presents with right upper quadrant abdominal pain. On examination he has peripheral oedema, ascites, and a pulsatile liver. On auscultation, he has a holo-systolic murmur along the left sternal border.

3. A 30-year-old man presents with chest pain and feeling faint. On examination, he has a pansystolic murmur and a fourth heart sound. ECG shows left ventricular hypertrophy. Echo shows septal hypertrophy and abnormal mitral valve motion.

4. A 40-year-old woman with Marfan's syndrome presents with shortness of breath, fainting spells, and pounding of the heart. On examination, she is noted to have capillary pulsation in the nail bed and pistol-shot femoral pulses. On auscultation she has a high-pitched diastolic murmur heard best at the lower left sternal edge.

5. A 40-year-old man presents after fainting during a work-out in the gym. On auscultation, he has a harsh mid-systolic crescendo-decrescendo systolic murmur in the aortic area radiating to the carotids.

Question 179
Theme: Diagnosis of traumatic injuries

Options:

A Pulmonary embolus	H Airway obstruction
B Fat embolism	I Cerebral injury
C Haemothorax	J Small bowel perforation
D Neurogenic shock	K Cardiac tamponade
E Cerebral compression	L Tension pneumothorax
F Perforated peptic ulcer	
G Haemobilia	

For each case below, choose the SINGLE most likely diagnosis from the above list of options. Each option may be used once, more than once, or not at all.

1. A 20-year-old man is thrown off his motorbike in an RTA and sustains an open femur fracture. He did not lose consciousness. On examination, he becomes confused and short of breath. He is noted to have cutaneous and mucous membrane petechiae.

2. A 25-year-old man presents with massive haematemesis. He has a stab wound in the right side of his chest. Endoscopy demonstrates clear oesophagus and stomach with gushing of blood in the duodenum and a drop in pulse.

3. A 20-year-old man is thrown out of his car in an RTA and arrives intubated with a large gaping temporal scalp wound. His BP is 80/50 with a pulse rate of 115. His pupils are equal and respond sluggishly. However he does not move his extremities. C-spine shows a fracture of C5. His chest is clear to auscultation and the abdomen is soft. He has no external signs of injury to his limbs. His CVP is 3.

4. A 30-year-old woman with severe maxillofacial injuries becomes confused and agitated.

5. A 20-year-old man is stabbed in the anterior left chest. He becomes dyspnoeic and hypotensive. On examination, he has distended neck veins and faint heart sounds. His pulse volume drops by greater than 10 mmHg with inspiration.

Question 180
Theme: The treatment of chest trauma

Options:

A	Exploratory laparotomy	I	CPR, adrenaline IV and intubate
B	Obtain portable chest X-ray		
C	Peritoneal lavage	J	Pericardiocentesis
D	Needle thoracocentesis	K	Atropine 1mg IV and intubate
E	Immediate thoracotomy of the left chest		
F	Thoracostomy tube insertion at the 9th ICS		
G	Immediate thoracotomy and simultaneous laparotomy in theatre		
H	Perform CPR and defibrillate		

For each case below, choose the SINGLE most appropriate form of treatment from the above list of options. Each option may be used once, more than once, or not at all.

1. A 20-year-old man is stabbed in the left axillary line at the 6th ICS. He has no breath sounds on the left. He has distended neck veins. His BP is 80/50.

2. A 30-year-old man is shot in the left axillary line at the 7th ICS. He has a thoracostomy tube inserted that drains 200 ml/hour of blood. The bleeding persists. Abdominal X-ray shows a bullet in the abdomen.

3. A 25-year-old man is shot in the left axillary line at the 7th ICS. He has no breath sounds on the left. A thoracostomy tube is inserted at the second ICS. No blood is drained. The BP drops even further.

4. A 28-year-old man is stabbed in the left chest under his nipple. His BP is 80/50 with a pulse rate of 120. He has distended neck veins. His BP drops to 70/50. He has vesicular breath sounds bilaterally.

5. A 30-year-old man is brought to Casualty after being stabbed in the left anterior chest. He collapses. ECG shows electro-mechanical dissociation with no pulse.

Question 181
Theme: The treatment of cardiac arrythmias

Options:

A	Atropine 1mg IV push	I	Lignocaine IV
B	Precordial thump	J	Morphine IM
C	CPR until a defibrillator is present		
D	CPR, adrenaline 1:1000 IV push		
E	Transvenous pacemaker		
F	Defibrillate at 200 Joules		
G	External pacemaker		
H	Oxygen 4 LPM		

For each patient below, choose the SINGLE most appropriate treatment from the above list of options. Each option may be used once, more than once, or not at all.

1. A 60-year-old man presents with chest pain and shortness of breath. His ECG shows sinus bradycardia of 45 beats/min.

2. A 55-year-old woman is noted to have a slow heart rate. She is asymptomatic. ECG shows no relation between atrial and ventricular rhythm. The ventricular rhythm is 40 beats/min. The QRS complex is wide.

3. A 60-year-old man collapses in the street. The event is un-witnessed. He has no pulse.

4. A 30-year-old man involved in a high speed RTA is found unconscious at the scene. He is breathing spontaneously. In Accident and Emergency, the ECG monitor now shows an irregular rhythm and no P, QRS, ST, or T waves. The rate is rapid.

5. A 50-year-old man presents to Casualty with severe chest pain. He has a history of angina. The pain is not relieved with GTN. His BP is 120/70 with a pulse rate of 100. His ECG shows regular sinus rhythm.

Question 182
Theme: The treatment of cardiac conditions

Options:

A	Anticoagulation and digitalisation	I	Start dopamine infusion
B	GTN	J	IV frusemide
C	Propranolol	K	Carotid sinus massage
D	Adrenaline		
E	Lignocaine		
F	DC conversion with 200 Joules		
G	Atropine		
H	Check digoxin level		

For each case below, choose the SINGLE most appropriate form of treatment from the above list of options. Each option may be used once, more than once, or not at all.

1. A 50-year-old man presents with shortness of breath. His pulse has an irregular rate and rhythm. The chest X-ray shows cardiomegaly and left atrial enlargement. ECG shows atrial fibrillation with a rate of 180.

2. A 60-year-old man is on verapamil for hypertension and digoxin for atrial fibrillation. He is listed for herniorrhaphy. His preoperative ECG shows inverted p waves after the QRS complex and a regular rhythm. He is asymptomatic.

3. A 70-year-old patient in ITU suddenly loses consciousness. His ECG shows ventricular tachycardia.

4. A 40-year-old man admitted for acute myocardial infarction suddenly drops his BP to 70/45. He has bilateral rales on auscultation of his lung fields.

5. A 50-year-old man in ITU is noted to have paroxysmal supraventricular tachycardia on his ECG monitor.

Question 183
Theme: The management of paediatric gastrointestinal disorders

Options:

A Vancomycin   I Loperamide
B Panproctocolectomy
C Gluten-free diet
D Pancreatic enzyme supplementation
E Barium enema
F Rectal biopsy
G D penicillamine and avoidance of chocolates, nuts and shellfish
H Diverting colostomy

For each case below, choose the SINGLE most appropriate management option from the above list of options. Each option may be used once, more than once, or not at all.

1. A 2-year-old girl presents with failure to thrive and diarrhoea. She is found to have iron deficiency anaemia. Small bowel biopsy shows flattened villi, elongated crypts, and loss of columnar cells.

2. A 12-year-old boy is being treated for osteomyelitis. He has been on intravenous antibiotics for 2 weeks. He now has diarrhoea. On sigmoidoscopy, there are multiple patchy yellowish areas of necrotic mucosa.

3. A 6-month-old baby boy presents with repeated bouts of vomiting and abdominal distention. He is normal between attacks. A sausage-shaped mass is palpated in his abdomen.

4. A 2-month-old baby girl presents with failure to thrive. She has frequent episodes of vomiting with abdominal distention. The abdominal X-ray shows proximal bowel dilatation and no faeces or gas in the rectum.

5. A 12-year-old boy presents with liver disease. A slit-lamp examination reveals Kayser-Fleischer rings in his cornea. His urinary copper level is high.

Question 184
Theme: The management of airway obstruction

Options:

A	Endotracheal intubation	I	Tracheostomy
B	IM adrenaline 1:1000	J	Oxygen and IV
C	Cricothyroidotomy		aminophylline
D	Oxygen 60% and salbutamol nebuliser		
E	Heimlich manoeuvre		
G	IV dexamethasone		
H	Adrenaline nebuliser		

For each patient below, choose the SINGLE most appropriate management option from the above list of options. Each option may be used once, more than once, or not at all.

1. A 10-year-old boy presents with a boiled sweet stuck in his throat. He is in respiratory distress and cyanotic.

2. A 5-year-old girl presents acutely with stridor. She is using her accessory muscles of respiration. She is distressed and tachypnoeic.

3. A 10-year-old boy with a history of asthma presents acutely with shortness of breath and expiratory wheezing. His respiratory rate is 30. On auscultation, he now has a silent chest.

4. A 25-year-old woman is brought to Casualty by ambulance having sustained gross maxillofacial deformities following a high speed RTA. She is now agitated and hypoxic.

5. A 20-year-old man collapses in the street. His wife states that he has been bothered by a sore throat recently. The paramedics arrive, assess his airway, attempt and fail intubation. He now has laryngeal spasm and is turning blue.

Question 185
Theme: The management of ENT emergencies

Options:

A	Give nifedipine 10 mg	I	Ligate sphenopalatine
B	Obtain a barium swallow		artery in theatre
C	Obtain a sialogram	J	Consult haematologist
D	Advise patient to drink more	K	Check INR
	fluids and avoid citrus fruits		
E	List for bronchoscopy		
F	List for rigid oesophagoscopy		
G	IM buscopan		
H	Insert two large bore intravenous		
	cannulas and run gelofusin		

For each patient below, choose the SINGLE most appropriate management option from the above list of options. Each option may be used once, more than once, or not at all.

1. A 70-year-old woman presents with severe epistaxis. Her BP is noted to be 205/115. She has no prior history of hypertension. She denies aspirin or warfarin use. Bloods are taken, and an intravenous line is inserted. She continues to bleed profusely through her nose packs.

2. A 60-year-old man on warfarin 6 mg od for a previous DVT now presents with right-sided epistaxis. His BP is 120/70 with a pulse rate of 90. He has no visible vessels in Little's area. He continues to bleed through the nose pack.

3. A 60-year-old woman presents with a piece of chicken stuck in her throat. Soft tissue neck X-ray reveals a calcified bolus at the level of the cricopharyngeus.

4. A 70-year-old woman complains of mashed potato stuck in her throat since dinner. She is not distressed. She is able to sip water.

5. A 30-year-old man complains of intermittent unilateral cheek swelling with eating. On examination, no swelling is palpated, and the oral cavity is clear.

Question 186
Theme: Organisms that cause infection

Options:

A	*Pseudomonas aeruginosa*	I	Campylobacter
B	*Escherichia coli*	J	*Streptococcus pneumoniae*
C	*Staphylococcus aureus*	K	Mycobacterium
D	*Clostridium difficile*	L	Mycoplasma
E	*Clostridium perfringens*		
F	*Yersinia enterocolitica*		
G	*Neisseria gonorrhoea*		
H	*Chlamydia trachomatis*		

For each case below, choose the SINGLE most likely cause from the above list of options. Each option may be used once, more than once, or not at all.

1. A 50-year-old man in ITU has remained intubated for 10 days. He is now pyrexial. He has diminished breath sounds. Swabs from the ventilator tubing show Gram-negative rods.

2. A 30-year-old woman complains of severe right lower quadrant pain and watery diarrhoea. She is pyrexial. She had visited her parents in the country a week ago.

3. A 20-year-old man presents with right knee pain and swelling not associated with trauma. Synovial fluid is aspirated and reveals many diplococci. He also admits to a creamy yellow penile discharge.

4. A 50-year-old diabetic man presents with a painful and swollen right leg. X-ray demonstrates air in the soft tissues.

5. A 40-year-old man complains of profuse watery diarrhoea after 2 weeks of antibiotic therapy. Sigmoidoscopy reveals yellow necrotic regions.

Question 187
Theme: Investigations of surgical disease

Options:

A   Gastrograffin swallow
B   Upright chest X-ray
C   Abdominal X-ray
D   Full blood count
E   Mesenteric arteriogram
F   Computed tomography of the abdomen
G   Technetium 99 radioactive scan
H   Abdominal ultrasound

I   Serum urea and electrolytes
J   Stool culture

For each case below, choose the SINGLE most discriminating investigation from the above list of options. Each option may be used once, more than once, or not at all.

1. A 60-year-old man, postop rigid oesophagoscopy and removal of a foreign body, now presents with substernal pain, fever and tachypnoea.

2. A 65-year-old man with a history of cirrhosis, presents with massive rectal bleeding, and right lower quadrant pain. NG tube lavage reveals no blood in the stomach. Colonoscopy reveals no varices. You suspect angiodysplasia of the caecum.

3. A 20-year-old man presents with passage of frank blood and clots from his rectum. His blood tests, barium enema, and upper GI series are all normal.

4. A 60-year-old man with lung cancer is noted to have elevated liver function tests. You suspect metastatic disease.

5. A 65-year-old alcoholic now presents with a tender, palpable midline mass. He was recently hospitalised for acute pancreatitis 2 weeks prior. He has a raised amylase. You now suspect he has a pancreatic pseudocyst.

Options:

- A   Skin prick testing
- B   Patch testing
- C   Serum IgE levels
- D   RAST
- E   Oral challenge testing
- F   Measure C1 and C4 levels
- G   IM adrenaline 1:1000 + piriton treatment
- H   Inspect for nasal polyps

For each case below, choose the SINGLE most discriminating investigation from the above list of options. Each option may be used once, more than once, or not at all.

1. A 30-year-old man presents with nasal blockage and watery nasal discharge. He states the symptoms are worse at work. The floors are carpeted, and there is central heating. On examination, he has oedematous and pale nasal inferior turbinates.

2. A 20-year-old female is started on penicillin for acute tonsillitis. She develops stridor and a generalised rash.

3. A 10-year-old boy presents with abdominal pain and bloating after eating shellfish.

4. A 12-year-old boy with cystic fibrosis complains of bilateral nasal blockage and mouth-breathing.

5. A 30-year-old woman presents with recurrent attacks of cutaneous swelling of her face. These episodes seem to be triggered by stress. There is no associated urticaria or pruritis.

Question 189
Theme: Diagnosis of ENT diseases

Options:

A	Malignant otitis externa	J	Glandular fever
B	Rhinocerebral mucormycosis		
C	Lymphoma		
D	Quinsy		
E	Nasal polyposis		
F	Rhinosinusitis		
G	Otitis externa		
H	Acute otitis media		
I	Otitis media with effusion		

For each patient below, choose the SINGLE most likely diagnosis from the above list of options. Each option may be used once, more than once, or not at all.

1. A 50-year-old poorly controlled diabetic woman presents with periorbital and perinasal swelling with bloody nasal discharge. On examination, the nasal mucosa is black and necrotic.

2. A 25-year-old man presents with worsening sore throat. On examination he has trismus and unilateral enlargement of his right tonsil.

3. A 60-year-old woman is noted to have unilateral tonsillar enlargement. She denies sore throat.

4. A 30-year-old woman complains of otalgia and purulent discharge from the right ear. On examination, the external auditory meatus is swollen, and the canal is inflamed and filled with a creamy white discharge.

5. A 60-year-old diabetic woman complains of severe otalgia. On examination, she has granulation tissue in her ear canal.

Question 190
Theme: Investigation of gastrointestinal disorders

Options:

A	Sigmoidoscopy and biopsy	I	Paracentesis
B	Barium enema	J	Full blood count
C	Abdominal X-ray	K	Liver function tests
D	Upright chest X-ray		
E	Abdominal ultrasound		
F	Abdominal CT scan		
G	Liver biopsy		
H	Endocervical smear and culture		

For each patient below, choose the most discriminating investigation from the above list of options. Each option may be used once, more than once, or not at all.

1. A 30-year-old female taking oral contraceptives presents to her GP complaining of right upper quadrant abdominal discomfort.

2. A 22-year-old female presents with fever and right upper quadrant abdominal pain. On pelvic examination, she has adnexal tenderness and purulent cervical discharge.

3. A 35-year-old obese female presents with fever, vomiting, and right upper quadrant abdominal pain. The pain is worse on inspiration.

4. A 50-year-old heavy drinker presents with fever, jaundice, ascites, and right upper quadrant pain. Blood tests reveal a leukocytosis, increased LFTs, and a raised serum bilirubin. Of note, the SGOT is higher than the SGPT.

5. A 20-year-old female presents with recurrent episodes of colicky abdominal pain and diarrhoea. On examination, she is also noted to have perianal fistulae.

Question 191
Theme: The management of dysfunctional uterine bleeding

Options:

A   Hysterectomy
B   Clomiphene citrate
C   Oral contraceptives
D   Measure progesterone level at day 21
E   Pipelle endometrial sampling
F   Ethinylestradiol
G   Mefenamic acid
H   Provera
I   Hysteroscopy

For each case below, choose the SINGLE most appropriate treatment from the above list of options. Each option may be used once, more than once, or not at all.

1. A 25-year-old married woman presents with irregular menstrual cycles and menorrhagia. She would not like to start a family yet.

2. A 50-year-old woman presents with abnormal uterine bleeding.

3. A 14-year-old female complains of heavy periods and pain. She is not sexually active.

4. A 35-year-old married woman presents with intermenstrual spotting. She would like to conceive.

5. A 33-year-old woman presents with intermenstrual bleeding that is not controlled with oral contraceptives.

Question 192
Theme: The treatment of dysmenorrhoea

Options:

- A   Laser treatment at laparoscopy
- B   Danazol
- C   Oral contraceptives
- D   Mefenamic acid (Ponstan)
- E   Gonadotrophin releasing hormone agonist (Soladex)
- F   Total abdominal or vaginal hysterectomy
- G   No treatment
- H   Pelvic sympathectomy
- I   Laparotomy

For each case below, choose the SINGLE most appropriate treatment option from the above list of options. Each option may be used once, more than once, or not at all.

1. A 30-year-old woman complains of painful periods and pain during intercourse. She is afebrile and has a firm, tender nodule into the pouch of Douglas. Small foci of endometriosis are found at the time of laparoscopy.

2. A 28-year-old woman is diagnosed with endometriosis. Her symptoms are not incapacitating. She would like to start a family.

3. A 45-year-old woman complains of intractable dysmenorrhoea and menorrhagia. She does not want any more children.

4. A 40-year-old woman is diagnosed with endometriosis. The pain is severe, and she refuses surgical treatment. She does not want any more children.

5. A 20-year-old woman presents with severe left lower abdominal pain, increasing abdominal girth, painful periods, and menorrhagia. Ultrasound demonstrates a 20 cm left ovarian cyst.

Question 193
Theme: Causes of painful or swollen ear

Options:

- A Subperichondrial haematoma
- B Perichondritis
- C Subperichondrial abscess
- D Acute mastoiditis
- E Keloid
- F Infected preauricular sinus
- G Malignant otitis externa
- H Acute otitis externa
- I Ramsay Hunt syndrome

For each case below, choose the SINGLE most likely cause from the above list of options. Each option may be used once, more than once, or not at all.

1. A 30-year-old rugby player presents with a swollen and painful upper pinna after being struck in the side of his head. On palpation, the swelling is boggy and tense.

2. A 70-year-old man is noted to have a collapsed pinna. He states he has had this for 15 years.

3. A 25-year-old woman presents with intermittent discharge and a swelling in front of her right ear.

4. A 60-year-old woman presents with unilateral left-sided hearing loss and a painful left ear. On examination, she has skin eruption vesicles in front of her ear.

5. A 12-year-old boy presents with a painful right ear. He is febrile. On examination, the pinna is pushed forwards and downwards. He is tender on palpation of the concha.

Question 194
Theme: The treatment of cardiac conditions

Options:

A   Oxygen, morphine and streptokinase therapy
B   Coronary artery vein bypass grafting
C   Angioplasty
D   Intra-aortic balloon pumping
E   Swan–Ganz catherisation
F   Defibrillation
G   Oxygen, IV frusemide, morphine and glyceryl trinitrate
H   GTN tablet and atenolol
I   GTN tablet and nifedipine

For each case below, choose the SINGLE most appropriate form of treatment from the above list of options. Each option may be used once, more than once, or not at all.

1. A 40-year-old man has severe mitral valve regurgitation and is unable to maintain an adequate cardiac output. He is awaiting a valve replacement.

2. A 50-year-old man presents with dyspnoea and tachycardia. He has bilateral rales on auscultation of his lung fields. He has a history of ischaemic heart disease. Chest X-ray shows cardiomegaly and pulmonary oedema.

3. A 60-year-old man complains of chest pain after jogging. He takes ventolin inhaler for his asthma. ECG shows ST segment depression.

4. A 55-year-old man with frequent episodes of angina, now complains that the pain is no longer alleviated on rest or with GTN. Coronary angiogram shows left main stem obstruction.

5. A 60-year-old man complains of severe excruciating chest pain at rest. He is diaphoretic and nauseous. The ECG shows Q waves and ST elevation in leads I, II and AVL.

Question 195
Theme: The treatment of abdominal pain

Options:

    A   ERCP and endoscopic sphincterotomy
    B   Laparoscopic cholecystectomy
    C   IV fluids, IV antibiotics and analgesia
    D   Subtotal colectomy, mucous fistula and permanent ileostomy
    E   Laparotomy
    F   Mesalazine
    G   Panproctocolectomy
    H   Hartmann's procedure

For each case below, choose the SINGLE most appropriate treatment from the above list of options. Each option may be used once, more than once, or not at all.

1. A 20-year-old female presents with recurrent bloody diarrhoea and crampy abdominal pain. Sigmoidoscopy and biopsy confirm ulcerative colitis.

2. A 25-year-old man involved in an RTA sustains blunt trauma to his upper abdomen. He complains of left shoulder pain and diffuse abdominal pain. He becomes increasingly tachycardic and hypotensive and develops peritoneal signs.

3. A 40-year-old woman presents with pyrexia and right upper quadrant abdominal pain. The white cell count is 14 with elevated neutrophils. Both the chest X-ray and the abdominal X-ray are unremarkable.

4. A 50-year-old man presents with fever, right upper quadrant pain, and jaundice. Ultrasound reveals a dilated common bile duct.

5. A 30-year-old man presents with severe, intractable abdominal pain. He is pyrexial, tachycardic, and has marked abdominal distension. On X-ray, the colon is noted to have a transverse diameter of 7 cm.

Question 196
Theme: Diagnosis of penile conditions

Options:

  A   Phimosis
  B   Paraphimosis
  C   Priapism
  D   Penile warts
  E   Peyronie's disease
  F   Squamous cell carcinoma of the penis
  G   Erythroplasia of Queyrat
  H   Impotence
  I   Balanitis xerotica obliterans

For each case below, choose the SINGLE most likely diagnosis from the above list of options. Each option may be used once, more than once, or not at all.

1. A 40-year-old man presents to Casualty with a painful penis. On examination, the foreskin is retracted behind the glans with glandular swelling.

2. A 12-year-old boy with a history of UTIs presents with difficulty urinating. On examination, the opening of the foreskin is pinhole in size.

3. A 50-year-old man with a history of chronic renal failure presents with a painful penis. On examination, the corpus cavernosa are erect, and the corpus spongiosum is flaccid.

4. A 40-year-old man with Riedel's thyroiditis complains that intercourse is painful. He provides a photo that shows dorsal curvature of the erect penis.

5. A 55-year-old man complains that he is unable to obtain an erection. He had undergone abdominal aortic aneurysm repair recently.

Question 197
Theme: Diagnosis of benign breast diseases

Options:

A	Breast abscess	J	Fat necrosis
B	Benign mammary dysplasia	K	Duct ectasia
C	Fibroadenoma	L	Ruptured breast implant
D	Periductal mastitis	M	Cystic disease
E	Silicon granulomas		
F	Leaking breast implant		
G	Sebaceous cyst		
H	Duct papilloma		
I	Lipoma		

For each case below, choose the SINGLE most likely diagnosis from the above list of options. Each option may be used once, more than once, or not at all.

1. A 33-year-old female is found to have rippling of the lower margins of her breast implants.

2. A 30-year-old female presents with a smooth, firm 3 cm breast mass that is not attached to skin. FNAC shows no malignant cells.

3. A 20-year-old female complains of breast lumpiness and breast pain prior to her periods. On examination, her breasts are tender in the outer quadrants with some nodularity. FNAC shows fibrosis, adenosis and cystic changes.

4. A 50-year-old woman presents with multiple discrete smooth breast lumps. Yellow fluid is obtained on aspiration. FNAC shows no malignant cells.

5. A 40-year-old woman presents with persistent cheesy nipple discharge. She is noted to have nipple retraction and no discrete lumps. Mammogram shows duct thickening.

Question 1: Answers

1. **A**
   Classic presentation for acute appendicitis.

2. **G**
   Gallstones and alcohol are the main predisposing factors for acute pancreatitis.

3. **H**
   Chronic active hepatitis is associated with methyldopa and also isoniazid.

4. **B**
   Chronic diverticular disease mimics colon cancer, but as the latter is not a listed option, chronic diverticular disease is the obvious diagnosis.

5. **J**

Question 2: Answers

1. **A**

2. **J**

3. **D**

4. **C**
   Chlamydia can be associated with adhesions particularly around the liver.

5. **B**

Question 3: Answers

1. **B**
   The presentation is one of hypoglycaemia.

2. C
Lumbar puncture is the investigation of choice for meningitis. However, intravenous antibiotic therapy should not be delayed to secure a diagnosis.

3. D

4. D

5. D

Question 4: Answers

1. A
The presentation fits Meniere's disease which requires recurrent episodes to make the diagnosis.

2. D
Both asymmetrical sensorineural hearing loss and unilateral tinnitus require a magnetic resonance (MR) scan of the internal acoustic meatus to exclude acoustic neuroma.

3. B

4. H
Whiplash affecting the cervical spine can be associated with vertigo as can head injury.

5. C

Question 5: Answers

1. A
This case of testicular torsion requires urgent surgical exploration.

2. E
This is a case of seminoma which classically spreads via the lymphatics to the paraaortic lymph nodes. This testicular tumour readily responds to radiotherapy.

3. **F**
This is a case of teratoma which is treated with cytotoxic drugs.

4. **G**
This is a case of acute epididymo-orchitis.

5. **H**
This is a case of an epididymal cyst and not a hydrocoele as the testis is palpable separately.

Question 6: Answers

1. **D**

2. **K**
D is also an option. However, K stresses the importance that an operation with expected blood loss cannot be denied to a Jehovah's Witness on the basis of his refusal to receive blood transfusion.

3. **J**

4. **F**

5. **H**

6. **A**

7. **N**

8. **C**

9. **C**

10. **L**

Question 7: Answers

1. **D**
This patient is suffering from Alzheimer's disease.

2. **K**

3. **A**
This patient exhibits suicidal thoughts, which is more than a grief reaction.

4. **E**

5. **G**
This patient shows signs of opiate abuse.

Question 8: Answers

1. **A**
Koplik's spots are seen prior to the measles rash.

2. **F**
This is a patient with glandular fever and upper airway obstruction.

3. **E**

4. **C**

5. **I**

Question 9: Answers

1. **A**

2. **J**

3. **E**

4. **B**

5. **F**

Question 10: Answers

1. **K**
This patient has Addison's disease.

2. G
This patient presents with classic signs and symptoms of hypothyroidism.

3. A
Viable protozoon cysts are ingested in contaminated food.

4. H
This patient presents with pancreatic cancer. Sudden onset of diabetes in the elderly is also suggestive.

5. I
Barium swallow followed by upper GI endoscopy are needed to exclude oesophageal pathology.

Question 11: Answers

1. H
Infectious mononucleosis is associated with hepatitis.

2. I
This is a case of subacute bacterial endocarditis.

3. D
Unilateral enlargement of the tonsil may either be associated with quinsy, lymphoma, or carcinoma. Fluctuating fever and the absence of pain suggest a diagnosis of lymphoma.

4. J
Typical features of sarcoidosis for which the Kveim test is diagnostic.

5. G
Scrofula is a sign of tuberculosis for which the Mantoux test is diagnostic.

Question 12: Answers

1. H
Children under 5 are at risk as they do not develop specific antibodies against *H. influenzae* until after the age of 5.

2. **D**
Tuberculous meningitis.

3. **A**
Meningococcal meningitis.

4. **K**
Viral meningitis

5. **I**
Oral rifampicin is the recognised prophylactic treatment for close contacts.

Question 13: Answers

1. **I**

2. **F**

3. **D**

4. **H**

5. **A**

Question 14: Answers

1. **F**
Between 1 and 5% of pregnant women will carry *Listeria monocytogenes* in the rectum. It can also be acquired from eating unpasteurised cheese and from cooked meats. Treatment is with ampicillin IV.

2. **C**
Microscopy with a drop of saline shows the flagellate organisms. Treatment is with oral metronidazole.

3. **H**
Treponema pallidum is extremely sensitive to penicillin.

4. **E**

Unfortunately acyclovir is not recommended during pregnancy. *Herpes neonatorum* produces a 20% mortality in infants.

5. **K**

Toxoplasmosis gondii is treated with spiromycin. It is transmitted through infected cat faeces.

Question 15: Answers

1. **K**

Postpartum haemorrhage requires loss of greater than 500 ml of blood.

2. **I**

3. **G**

The presence of amniotic fluid is consistent with rupture of membranes.

4. **C**

5. **B**

Question 16: Answers

1. **F**

Axillary lymphadenopathy is indicative of malignancy.

2. **B**

3. **E**

4. **J**

Paget's disease or intraductal carcinoma is associated with eczema of the nipple especially in the presence of a firm nodule suggestive of more than simple eczema.

5. **H**

Question 17: Answers

1. I

2. D
A thyroglossal cyst moves on swallowing or protrusion of the tongue. The fact that the swelling transilluminates excludes a thyroid swelling.

3. F

4. A

5. B
Ludwig's angina, a submandibular abscess, usually arises from an abscess of the lower premolars or the first and second molar.

Question 18: Answers

1. C

2. J

3. D
Pernicious anaemia is also associated with antibodies to parietal cells.

4. A
Alcoholism is more associated with vitamin B_1 and folate deficiency. Here gastrectomy is the aetiology of the vitamin B_{12} deficiency.

5. I
Heinz bodies are associated with G6PDD.

Question 19: Answers

1. F

2. A

3. H

4. I

5. A

Question 20: Answers

1. **A**
A rodent ulcer is associated with BCC. BCC also has a predilection for the pinna.

2. **D**
Rubber (aromatic amines) is associated with bladder carcinoma.

3. **I**
Coeliac disease is a risk factor for lymphoma of the small bowel.

4. **H**
Although SCC can present on the lower lip, alcohol and betel nut chewing are risk factors associated more with oral cancer which can also present on the lower lip.

5. **F**
Asbestosis and tobacco are recognised risk factors for bronchial carcinoma.

Question 21: Answers

1. H

2. B

3. C

4. G

5. I

Question 22: Answers

1. **J**
   Rheumatoid arthritis.

2. **F**
   Myasthenia gravis.

3. **A**
   Systemic lupus erythematosus.

4. **G**
   Wegener's granulomatosis.

5. **B**
   Pernicious anaemia.

Question 23: Answers

1. **J**

2. **I**

3. **A**

4. **K**

5. **D**

Question 24: Answers

1. **F**

2. **E**
   Stress incontinence.

3. **C**

4. **H**
   Benign prostatic hypertrophy.

5. **A**
Urinary tract infection.

Question 25: Answers

1. D

2. I

3. G

4. H

5. C

Question 26: Answers

1. **B**
Chvostek's sign is demonstrated here and is associated with hypocalcaemia.

2. **A**
Upright chest X-ray looking for free air under the diaphragm to exclude perforated peptic ulcer disease is suggested here.

3. **J**
Blood loss from a hip fracture often warrants blood replacement.

4. **H**
Pulmonary embolism is suggested here.

5. **I**
Epidural anaesthesia may be associated with urinary retention.

Question 27: Answers

1. A

2. D

3. C

4. B

5. C

Question 28: Answers

1. K
Pretibial myxoedema is associated with hyperthyroidism.

2. H
Necrobiosis lipoidica is associated with diabetes mellitus.

3. I
Dermatitis herpetiformis is associated with coeliac disease.

4. F
Erythema multiforme may be associated with Stevens–Johnson syndrome.

5. B

Question 29: Answers

1. H

2. E

3. G

4. C

5. B

Question 30: Answers

1. L

2. K

3. E

4. C

5. D

Question 31: Answers

1. K

2. C

3. E

4. G

5. I

Question 32: Answers

1. I

   Phytomenadione or vitamin K is required. Means of administration depend on the patient's need for anticoagulation as
   intravenous vitamin K is erratic and may normalise the INR
   rapidly.

2. B

   N-acetylcysteine is the antidote for paracetamol poisoning.
   Coproxamol contains paracetamol and dextropropoyxphene
   HCL.

3. G

4. K

5. H

Question 33: Answers

1. I

2. D

3. F

4. G

5. E

Question 34: Answers

1. A

2. B

3. H

4. I

5. E

Question 35: Answers

1. L

2. C

3. F

4. A

5. G

Question 36: Answers

1. K
The T wave changes in V5 and V6 suggest a lateral component to the inferior MI.

2. C
Atrial fibrillation may be associated with hyperthyroidism.

3. F

4. **H**
Hypokalaemia is a recognised complication of diuretic use.

5. **G**

Question 37: Answers

1. **I**
The diagnosis is likely to be hyperthyroidism.

2. **F**
Meningococcal meningitis is the most likely cause for this girl's collapse.

3. **K**

4. **A**

5. **C**
An urgent CT scan is required to exclude intracranial haemorrhage.

Question 38: Answers

1. **H**
The presentation is suggestive of ureteric colic.

2. **I**
The presentation is suggestive of ovarian cyst.

3. **C**
The presentation is suggestive of peptic ulcer disease.

4. **A**
The presentation is suggestive of abdominal aortic aneurysm. The size should be evaluated by ultrasound and surgical repair is advisable if the aneurysm is greater than 5 cm in diameter.

5. **K**
Steroid usage for rheumatoid arthritis puts this woman at risk for a perforated peptic ulcer.

Question 39: Answers

1. K

2. F

3. A

4. C

5. D

Question 40: Answers

1. A
   Topical tar is the treatment of choice for psoriasis.

2. B
   Topical steroids is the treatment of choice for eczema.

3. K
   Oral nystatin is the treatment of choice for oral candidiasis.

4. F
   Oral prednisolone is the treatment of choice for pemphigus vulgaris. This condition may be precipitated by penicillamine.

5. B
   Contact dermatitis is treated with topical steroids and avoidance.

Question 41: Answers

1. B

2. G

3. A

4. C

5. F

Question 42: Answers

1. C

2. E

3. B

4. I

5. G

Question 43: Answers

1. C
    Cold haemagglutinins are associated with 50% of untreated *Mycoplasma pneumoniae* infection and a titre of 1:64 supports the diagnosis.

2. J

3. A

4. B

5. F

Question 44: Answers

1. H
    Proctosigmoidoscopy and biopsy are suggested for Crohn's disease.

2. I
    This patient most likely has Cushing's disease.

3. C
    This patient most likely has Addison's disease.

4. B
    This patient most likely has hypothyroidism.

5. F
This patient is likely to be a new-onset diabetic.

Question 45: Answers

1. K
Weight loss and salt restriction are advocated initially.

2. A

3. B
As this patient is an asthmatic, beta blocker therapy is contra-indicated.

4. I

5. E

Question 46: Answers

1. D

2. C

3. I
Pneumocystis carinii is treated with pentamidine.

4. F
Sarcoidosis is treated with steroid therapy.

5. G
Tuberculosis is treated with multiple antituberculous chemo-therapy.

Question 47: Answers

1. A
Presbyacusis is confirmed by pure tone audiogram which would demonstrate symmetrical high frequency sensorineural hearing loss.

2. D
Syringing, cotton bud usage, and swimming are recognised risk factors for otitis externa.

3. I
A conductive hearing loss with a normal tympanic membrane is suggestive of otosclerosis.

4. E
Chronic secretory otitis media or glue ear is treated with watchful waiting for 3 months. If spontaneous resolution has not occurred, referral to an ENT specialist may be necessary.

5. H
This patient has a false negative Rinne test suggestive of dead ear.

Question 48: Answers

1. A
Flucloxacillin is associated with cholestatic jaundice.

2. E
High bilirubin on fasting is diagnostic of Gilbert's syndrome, an inherited metabolic disorder leading to increased unconjugated hyperbilirubinaemia.

3. F
Chronic active hepatitis or specifically lupoid CAH presents in young females with inflammation of the liver for at least 3–6 months.

4. J
Primary biliary cirrhosis is a progressive non-suppurative cholangiohepatitis with destruction of the small interlobular bile ducts.

5. B
The presentation is one of hepatitis A which can be acquired through the fecal-oral route. Methyldopa is associated with haemolytic jaundice and would not present with signs of obstructive jaundice as in this case.

Question 49: Answers

1. **K**
   Gonococcal arthritis has a predilection for upper extremity joints. This helps differentiate between Reiter's syndrome, which predominantly affects the lower extremity joints.

2. **F**
   The triad of symptoms are classic for Reiter's syndrome, one of the spondyloarthritides.

3. **I**
   Osteoarthritis is also associated with Heberden nodes of the DIP joints.

4. **E**

5. **C**
   Psoriatic arthropathy also has a predilection for the upper extremity joints. It can present in the toes and fingers as sausage digits. However, the skin and nail changes help to differentiate this condition from gout or rheumatoid arthritis.

Question 50: Answers

1. **F**
   Chronic renal failure.

2. **E**
   Hypercalcaemia associated with bone metastases.

3. **C**
   Chronic adrenal insufficiency.

4. **H**
   Acute intermittent porphyria from ingestion of the oral contraceptive pill.

5. **B**
   Perforated peptic ulcer with peritoneal signs.

Question 51: Answers

1. I

2. D

3. G

4. E

5. B

Question 52: Answers

1. **H**
   Miosis is a sign of opioid toxicity.

2. **A**
   Cefotaxime IV is appropriate treatment for meningococcal meninigitis in penicillin allergic patients.

3. **B**
   Contrast agents can precipitate pheochromocytoma hypertensive crises.

4. **G**
   Subdural haemorrhage is associated with alcoholics and epileptics who may not recall head trauma.

5. **C**
   This is a case of myxoedema.

Question 53: Answers

1. A

2. E

3. K

4. F

5. H

Question 54: Answers

1. G

2. C

3. B

4. J

5. I

Question 55: Answers

1. J
   Leptospirosis (Weil's disease) is a spirochaete transmitted in water infected by rat urine.

2. F
   Kala-azar or leishmaniasis is spread through the lymphatics through a cutaneous lesion.

3. G

4. B

5. I
   Felty's syndrome is the triad of rheumatoid arthritis, spleno-megaly, and leucopenia.

Question 56: Answers

1. H

2. K

3. C

4. A

5. E

Question 57: Answers

1. K

2. F

3. B

4. A

5. D

Question 58: Answers

1. K

2. E

3. I

4. H

5. G

Question 59: Answers

1. D

2. K

3. C

4. E

5. F

Question 60: Answers

1. H

2. G
   Solar keratosis is a premalignant condition.

3. F

4. C
   Café au lait patches are associated with neurofibromatosis.

5. B
   Acral lentiginous melanoma is often mistaken for subungual haematoma or chronic paronychia. The condition can also present as expanding areas of brown or black pigmentation on the palms or soles.

Question 61: Answers

1. G

2. F

3. D

4. H

5. A

Question 62: Answers

1. C

2. I

3. B

4. J

5. H

Question 63: Answers

1. **A**
Hypokalaemia is associated with the use of loop diuretics.

2. **H**
Convex elevation is suggestive of MI. Here the elevation is concave which is associated with pericarditis.

3. **G**
A diagnosis of inferior MI requires a Q wave in lead II also.

4. **C**
Hypocalcaemia is a recognised complication of thyroidectomy.

5. **J**
Classic for myxoedema.

Question 64: Answers

1. **I**
Courvoisier's law states that, 'if in a case of painless jaundice, the gallbladder is palpable, the cause will not be gallstones'.

2. **K**

3. **A**
Acute appendicitis is less likely without nausea and Crohn's ileitis is less likely without diarrhoea.

4. **G**
Carcinoma of the caecum is associated with bleeding.

5. **E**
The commonest presentation of carcinoma of the sigmoid is changes in bowel habit rather than pain.

Question 65: Answers

1. **B**
Cystic fibrosis is diagnosed by an abnormally high sweat chloride level.

2. **A**

Coeliac disease is suggested by a mixed anaemia (iron and folic acid deficiencies). However, the definitive diagnosis is made by biopsy of the jejunum.

3. **F**

This is a case of hyperthyroidism.

4. **J**

This is a case of juvenile onset diabetes mellitus.

5. **I**

The four classic signs of congestive heart failure include tachycardia, tachypnoea, cardiomegaly, and hepatomegaly.

Question 66: Answers

1. **F**

Battle's sign and blood in the ear canal is suggestive of a temporal bone fracture. Non-accidental injury should be considered.

2. **E**

Reye's syndrome can be precipitated by aspirin ingestion and presents with hepatomegaly and emesis.

3. **C**

This is a case of diabetic ketoacidosis.

4. **F**

Lumbar puncture should not be performed in the presence of papilloedema or other signs of increased intracranial pressure. Pathology may include brain tumours, brain abscess, intracranial bleed, etc.

5. **H**

Infants do not display classic signs for meningitis. However a full anterior fontanelle or opisthotonus (hyperextension of the spine) may aid in the diagnosis.

Question 67: Answers

1. **C**
The diagnosis is one of Alzheimer's dementia.

2. **D**
Idiopathic Parkinson's disease results from a progressive degeneration of the pigment-containing cells of the substantia nigra. This leads to dopamine deficiency.

3. **F**
Haloperidol is used to treat the tics in Gilles-de-la-Tourette syndrome.

4. **G**
The chorea in Huntington's chorea is controlled with tetrabenazine.

5. **J**
The patient is exhibiting signs of opioid withdrawal.

Question 68: Answers

1. **K**

2. **J**

3. **C**

4. **A**

5. **F**
A small skin tag or sentinel tag may be found at the lower end of a fissure-in-ano.

Question 69: Answers

1. **E**
Rectal disease is present in 30% of patients with ulcerative colitis.

2. **G**

3. **J**

4. **F**
Although diverticular disease is the most likely diagnosis, one must exclude carcinoma and adenoma.

5. **C**
90% of rectal carcinoma can be palpated by digital rectal exam.

Question 70: Answers

1. **A**
Anaphylaxis is treated with a prompt injection of 1 ml of 1:1000 adrenaline intramuscularly. This may need to be repeated.

2. **C**
Tension pneumothorax requires emergency needle decompression.

3. **D**
Cardiac tamponade requires swift needle pericardiocentesis.

4. **H**
This woman presents with a postoperative haematoma that needs urgent drainage, as it is now compressing her trachea.

5. **I**
This woman is at risk for a deep venous thrombosis and pulmonary embolism. Occasionally the signs of deep venous thrombosis appear after the pulmonary embolism which can make diagnosis difficult.

Question 71: Answers

1. **M**

2. **G**
Peutz–Jegher syndrome is melanosis of the lips and mucosa associated with jejunal polyposis.

3. **H**
   Fanconi's syndrome is an autosomal recessive renal tubular disorder that presents with rickets, glycosuria, phosphaturia, and aminoaciduria.

4. **D**

5. **L**
   Sjögren's syndrome presents here with rheumatoid arthritis, keratoconjunctivitis sicca and xerostomia.

Question 72: Answers

1. **G**
   Thiazide diuretics potentiate lithium toxicity.

2. **I**
   Cimetidine or tagamet potentiates warfarin toxicity as do aspirin, allopurinol, alcohol, disulfiram, erythromycin and a host of other drugs.

3. **E**
   Erythromycin potentiates carbamazepine toxicity as do isoniazid and verapamil.

4. **I**
   Cimetidine or tagamet potentiates the effects of phenytoin as do chloramphenicol, disulfiram and isoniazid.

5. **D**
   Alcohol is the culprit in this particular case.

Question 73: Answers

1. **I**

2. **B**

3. **A**

4. **D**

5. **G**

Question 74: Answers

1. J

2. C

3. G

4. H

5. D

Question 75: Answers

1. E

2. A

3. C

4. G

5. H
   The fine, wart-like lesions are better known as adenoma sebaceum which is commonly associated with tuberous sclerosis. Other skin lesions associated with this condition include areas of ash-leaf like hypopigmented spots over the trunk and limbs.

Question 76: Answers

1. F
   This baby is exhibiting typical features of cretinism.

2. H
   This newborn has adrenal hyperplasia and excessive production of androgens.

3. L
   The likely diagnosis is one of Cushing's syndrome from long-term steroid administration.

4. G
Galactosaemia arises from milk ingestion. The treatment is to avoid lactose in the diet.

5. C
This boy is suffering from diabetes insipidus.

Question 77: Answers

1. J
Alpha-1-antrypsin deficiency is often associated with emphysema and liver disease. Liver biopsy gives a definitive diagnosis.

2. A
Primary biliary cirrhosis is associated with hepatomegaly and a high alkaline phosphatase. Antibodies to mitochondria (AMA) are found in 95% of cases.

3. B
The classic triad for idiopathic haemochromatosis is bronze skin pigmentation, diabetes mellitus, and hepatomegaly.

4. C
Kayser–Fleischer rings are a specific sign for Wilson's disease, a rare inborn error of copper metabolism that leads to a failure of copper excretion.

5. G
This combination of autoimmune disease and hepatitis is suggestive of autoimmune chronic active hepatitis.

Question 78: Answers

1. H
Acute lumbar disc prolapse occurs most commonly at L5/S1.

2. J
Spinal stenosis is treated by surgical decompression.

3. A
Multiple myeloma is suggestive with a high ESR. Diagnosis is confirmed by the presence of paraprotein in the serum,

Bence–Jones protein in the urine and by the presence of lytic bone lesions.

4. **K**
Complications of Paget's disease include deafness, high-output cardiac failure, and osteogenic sarcoma.

5. **D**
Fusion of the sacroiliac joints is a common feature of ankylosing spondylitis.

Question 79: Answers

1. **F**
This is a case of lower motor neuron bladder neuropathy.

2. **A**
Excretion urography is useful to investigate the presence of renal disease predisposing to recurrent calculi formation.

3. **C**
Dynamic scintigraphy is used to assess renal blood flow, and in this case it is used to establish the extent of renal perfusion post transplantation.

4. **A**
An intravenous urogram will give evidence of renal function in benign prostatic hypertrophy. It may show hydronephrosis, bladder enlargement with chronic retention, or intravesical enlargement of the prostate.

5. **A**
In retroperitoneal fibrosis, excretion urography allows demonstration of obstruction to the ureter commencing at the level of the pelvic brim. Retroperitoneal fibrosis may be associated with retroperitoneal lymphoma, abdominal aortic aneurysm, and carcinoma of the bladder and colon.

Question 80: Answers

1. **K**
This multisystem disorder of thrombosis of microvasculature with acute glomerulonephritis is the most common cause of childhood acute renal failure.

2. **L**
   Acute tubulo-interstitial nephritis occurs most commonly as a hypersensitivity reaction to allopurinol, penicillins, NSAIDs, phenindione and sulphonamides.

3. **B**
   Amyloidosis is a disorder of protein metabolism. Patients can present with heart failure, nephrotic syndrome, or bleeding. Congo red stains the deposits of amyloid pink. Biopsies are taken from the gums or rectum.

4. **E**
   Wegener's granulomatosis is a generalised vasculitis that involves the upper respiratory tract, lungs and kidneys.

5. **A**
   Goodpasture's syndrome is a proliferative glomerulonephritis associated with recurrent haemoptysis.

Question 81: Answers

1. **E**
   The treatment for Goodpasture's syndrome is plasmapharesis and aggressive immunosuppressive therapy. Prognosis is poor.

2. **A**
   The treatment for Wegener's granulomatosis is cyclophosphamide.

3. **G**
   Dialysis is warranted here in view of the progressive uraemia. The history of heart disease and previous bowel surgery are soft contraindications to haemodialysis and peritoneal dialysis.

4. **L**
   Nephrotic syndrome most likely due to minimal change glomerulonephritis is managed here with a short course of prednisolone.

5. **F**
   Acute nephritic syndrome most likely due to post-streptococcal glomerulonephritis can be managed with conservative treatment with fluid and protein restriction. Penicillin is given for 3 months to reduce the risk of recurrence.

Question 82: Answers

1. A

2. B

3. H

4. I

5. K

Question 83: Answers

1. D
   Bouchard's nodes and 'poor man's gout' are signs of osteo-arthritis.

2. G

3. H

4. E

5. A
   Postoperative arthritis is usually due to gout.

Question 84: Answers

1. H

2. E

3. F

4. J

5. I

Question 85: Answers

1. B

2. C

3. F

4. I

5. G

Question 86: Answers

1. B

2. G
   Longitudinal temporal bone fractures are not classically associated with facial nerve injury and usually present with blood in the external auditory meatus and not haemotympanum.

3. C
   Ramsay Hunt disease is due to the Herpes zoster virus.

4. L

5. D

Question 87: Answers

1. A
   Budd–Chiari syndrome results from thrombosis of the major hepatic veins and is associated with the contraceptive pill.

2. J
   Bronzed diabetes or haemochromatosis is an autosomal recessive error of metabolism. Women present later as menstruation reduces the iron load.

3. **B**
Chlorpromazine is associated with obstructive jaundice.

4. **I**
Gamma-glutamyl transpeptidase is specific for alcoholic hepatitis.

5. **L**

Question 88: Answers

1. **L**

2. **J**

3. **K**

4. **H**

5. **F**
Tricuspid regurgitation is associated with endocarditis in drug addicts.

Question 89: Answers

1. **G**
This is a case of Takayasu's syndrome involving the subclavian arteries. Diagnosis is confirmed by angiogram.

2. **I**
Thromboangiitis obliterans or Buerger's disease is associated with young male smokers and often necessitates amputation for severe rest pain and ulceration as patients are unable to give up smoking.

3. **D**

4. **B**

5. **A**

Question 90: Answers

1. **A**

2. **H**
   Spontaneous pneumothorax occurs from a rupture of an apical pleural bleb and is associated with tall, young males and also with aeroplane ascent.

3. **E**
   Pulmonary embolism can present without the classic S1Q3T3 ECG strain pattern. Leg findings may also present later and not initially.

4. **C**
   Angina is aggravated by cold, by anxiety, and by exercise. In the case of a normal resting ECG, an exercise ECG should be obtained.

5. **L**
   Ovarian carcinoma can be associated with a right-sided pleural effusion (Meig's syndrome).

Question 91: Answers

1. **E**
   Wernicke–Korsakoff syndrome should be promptly treated with thiamine.

2. **D**
   Isoniazid is associated with Vitamin B_6 deficiency.

3. **L**
   This is a case of cocaine intoxication. Cocaine sniffing is associated with nasal septal perforation.

4. **M**
   Sinusitis, ear infections, skull fracture, etc. are risk factors for brain abscess.

5. **H**
   This is a case of delirium tremens.

Question 92: Answers

1. A
This is transmitted via inhalation from infected parrots.

2. M

3. H

4. I

5. E

Question 93: Answers

1. E
Bilateral internuclear ophthalmoplegia is almost pathognomonic for multiple sclerosis.

2. H
The Argyll Robertson pupil is almost pathognomonic for neurosyphilis. As her fasting blood glucose is normal, diabetes is excluded as a cause.

3. G

4. L

5. K
Oculomotor nerve lesion with sparing of the pupil is seen with infarction of the oculomotor nerve in diabetes. 'Sparing of the pupil' means the parasympathetic fibres which run on the superior surface of the nerve are spared.

Question 94: Answers

1. C

2. A

3. F

4. G

5. I
Acute intermittent porphyria is known to be precipitated by oral contraceptives. Other signs include peripheral motor neuropathy.

Question 95: Answers

1. B
Hypoparathyroidism may occur following thyroid or neck surgery.

2. K

3. I
This is a case of subdural haemorrhage. The elderly and epileptics are at risk. Head trauma may have gone unnoticed.

4. L
The purple papules are most likely Kaposi's sarcoma associated with HIV.

5. J
This is a case of hypoglycaemia. Binge drinking and poor nutrition are risk factors.

Question 96: Answers

1. C
Beck's triad consists of muffled heart sounds, hypotension, and Kussmaul's sign and is pathognomonic for cardiac tamponade.

2. G

3. M
Absence of the psoas shadow is due to retroperitoneal fluid.

4. I

5. K
Addisonian crisis is precipitated here by omission of doses of a long-term steroid regime.

Question 97: Answers

1. **K**
   Octreotide, a synthetic analogue of somatostatin (GHIRH) is the treatment of choice for acromegaly.

2. **J**
   Hypothyroidism is treated with daily thyroxine replacement.

3. **I**
   Propylthiouracil is not contraindicated during pregnancy for treatment of hyperthyroidism.

4. **E**
   Metyrapone, an 11-hydroxylase blocker, is the treatment of choice for Cushing's syndrome.

5. **F**
   Primary hypoadrenalism is treated with replacement of glucocorticoids and mineralocorticoids.

Question 98: Answers

1. **D**
   Patch testing for contact dermatitis may be useful. Otherwise treatment with topical corticosteroids should control this self-limiting condition.

2. **C**
   Wood's light produces a greenish fluorescence of the scalp when infected by *Microsporum canis*, the culprit behind tinea capitis.

3. **H**
   A photosensitive butterfly-distribution rash can be a presenting sign for systemic lupus erythematosus.

4. **A**
   Tinea cruris is treated with griseofulvin and local antifungal cream.

5. **G**
   Bullous pemphigoid is a disease of the elderly. Diagnosis is confirmed by the immunofluorescent staining of the basement membrane with IgG.

Question 99: Answers

1. A

2. C
   Malabsorption of fat can lead to vitamin K deficiency, a fat-soluble vitamin.

3. F
   Cheilosis or fissuring of the angles of the mouth is associated with riboflavin deficiency.

4. G
   Pellegra is associated with carcinoid syndrome because carcinoid tumour consumes tryptophan, nicotinamide's precursor.

5. L

Question 100: Answers

1. C

2. D
   Lateral medullary syndrome is caused by occlusion of the posterior inferior cerebellar artery or one vertebral artery leading to infarction of the lateral medulla and inferior surface of the cerebellum.

3. J

4. B

5. F

Question 101: Answers

1. D
   'Drop' attacks are commonly seen with vertebrobasilar ischaemia.

2. **A**
This is a case of hypoglycaemia.

3. **F**
This is a case of hypocalcaemia.

4. **B**
This is possibly a case of Stokes–Adams attack.

5. **I**
Postural hypotension is common in the elderly and is also a side-effect of levodopa.

Question 102: Answers

1. **B**
This is a case of alcoholic-induced hypoglycaemia.

2. **D**
Uraemia can arise from tetracycline administration in patients with poor renal function. Tetracycline has an antianabolic effect and leads to the buildup of nitrogenous waste products.

3. **L**
Petit mal seizures give the classic 3/second spike and wave activity on electroencephalogram.

4. **H**
Meningitis is investigated by CSF analysis from a lumbar puncture.

5. **N**
Patients with systemic lupus erythematosus have high titres of anti-double-stranded DNA.

Question 103: Answers

1. **E**
Patients with cystic fibrosis are at risk of pneumonia due to pseudomonas aeruginosa. Tobramycin is nephrotoxic and therefore, ciprofloxacin is a wiser choice.

2. **C**
Legionella pneumophila is transmitted through the cooling system or shower facilities associated with institutions.

3. **A**
Asthma may be managed initially with a salbutamol inhaler.

4. **I**
Cyclophosphamide is the treatment for Wegener's granulomatosis.

5. **H**
Farmer's lung or extrinsic allergic alveolitis is caused by inhalation of the spores of *Micropolyspora faeni*, found in mouldy hay.

Question 104: Answers

1. **F**
Migraine headaches can be treated with ergotamine, pizotifen (serotonin antagonist), or beta blockers. In this instance, pizotifen is the only drug that is not contraindicated in view of her other medical ailments.

2. **E**
Cluster headaches usually respond to ergotamine.

3. **J**
Acute sinusitis is treated by a course of antibiotics and a nasal decongestant.

4. **A**
Giant cell arteritis is treated promptly with prednisolone to avoid sudden blindness.

5. **H**
Trigeminal neuralgia is treated with carbamazepine.

Question 105: Answers

1. **M**
The common peroneal nerve can be damaged at the level of the fibular neck.

2. **D**
   Long thoracic nerve injury can also give a winged scapula but this does not disappear on forward thrusting of the shoulder.

3. **G**
   In ulnar nerve lesions the hand assumes the classic claw hand deformity.

4. **H**
   The pointing sign is associated with a median nerve injury.

5. **J**
   Injury to the sciatic nerve is assumed to occur from direct trauma or thermal injury from extruded acrylic cement.

Question 106: Answers

1. **B**

2. **D**

3. **K**

4. **F**

5. **I**

Question 107: Answers

1. **A**
   The Ortolani test is one of the tests for CDH.

2. **H**

3. **J**
   The normal angle is 160 degrees at birth and decreases to 125 degrees in adulthood.

4. **C**

5. **K**

Question 108: Answers

1. **J**
   Simmonds' test is demonstrated here.

2. **K**
   Charcot's joint, peripheral vascular disease, and osteoporosis are typical features of the diabetic foot.

3. **G**

4. **D**

5. **A**

Question 109: Answers

1. **A**

2. **C**

3. **F**

4. **H**

5. **K**

Question 110: Answers

1. **B**
   In a fit man under 60, AO cannulated screws are preferable to an Austin Moore hemiarthroplasty.

2. **F**
   Anterior cruciate ligament injury should be repaired surgically especially in a young athlete.

3. **I**
   Dynamic hip screw is the standard treatment for inter-trochanteric fractures.

4. D
Scapholunate disassociation is repaired by open reduction of the subluxation and a K wire to hold the reduction. The wrist is then splinted.

5. K
Anterior shoulder fracture-dislocation requires open reduction and fixation.

Question 111: Answers

1. G
Posterior shoulder dislocation is treated as detailed in option G.

2. A
Undisplaced supracondylar fractures are managed in children with a sling worn for 2–3 weeks.

3. H
Smith's fracture is the opposite of Colles' fracture and is treated by traction and extension of the wrist and cast immobilisation of the forearm for 6 weeks.

4. A
The pulled elbow is managed by wearing a sling for a few days for spontaneous recovery of the subluxation of the orbicular ligament which has slipped up over the head of the radius into the radiocapitellar joint. An alternative means of management is to forcefully supinate and flex the elbow.

5. E

Question 112: Answers

1. H
Metastases in the lungs precludes surgical treatment for osteosarcoma. X-ray findings describe Codman's triangle associated with osteosarcoma.

2. E
Spinal stenosis is treated surgical when the condition debilitates the patient.

3. **G**
Paget's disease of the bone is treated with calcitonin given subcutaneously or intramuscularly. Deafness is due to involvement of the bony foramina of the auditory nerve.

4. **H**
Multiple myeloma is treated with chemotherapy and supportive management.

5. **J**
Osteoid osteoma is treated by excision of the nidus in a small block of bone.

Question 113: Answers

1. **A**
Right hemicolectomy is the operation of choice for caecal volvulus causing large bowel obstruction.

2. **F**
Anterior resection is the operation of choice for rectal carcinomas that do not involve the anus.

3. **B**
An incarcerated irreducible inguinal hernia necessitates urgent herniorrhaphy.

4. **G**
Exploratory laparotomy is indicated for peritonitis and may require a Hartmann's procedure for diverticulitis or perforated carcinoma of the sigmoid.

5. **E**
Hartmann's procedure is an alternative.

Question 114: Answers

1. **I**
Anterior tibial compartment syndrome may be associated with severe exercise.

2. **B**
This patient also exhibits signs of venous insufficiency.

3. **E**

A mural thrombus following an MI, atrial fibrillation, or aneurysm may act as an embolic source.

4. **C**

Leriche's syndrome is buttock and thigh claudication with or without impotence and is a sign of aorto-iliac disease.

5. **D**

Question 115: Answers

1. **E**

Lower oesophageal or Schatzki's ring is treated with reassurance.

2. **A**

Monilial oesophagitis is treated with antifungal therapy. Immunosuppressed and patients with AIDS are at risk.

3. **B**

Quinsy is initially treated with incision and drainage followed by antibiotic therapy.

4. **G**

Ludwig's angina is treated with intravenous antibiotics.

5. **I**

Achalasia is treated with repeated dilatations. Heller's cardio-myotomy is reserved for failed cases.

Question 116: Answers

1. **A**

2. **C**

Mitral valve prolapse, scoliosis, myopia, and hypermobile joints are all characteristic of Marfan's syndrome.

3. **H**

Homocystinuria also presents in a similar fashion to Marfan's, however the former is associated with mental retardation. Here vascular thrombosis has resulted in a childhood MI.

4. **G**
   Hurler syndrome is one of the mucopolysaccharide disorders.

5. **E**
   Turner's syndrome is associated with lack of secondary sexual characteristics and with aortic stenosis and pigmented naevi.

Question 117: Answers

1. **J**
   Heimlich manouevre is essential to expel the foreign body from the trachea. Under non-emergency conditions, bronchoscopy is employed to remove the object.

2. **B**

3. **H**
   The child has acute epiglottitis. Complete airway obstruction from a swollen epiglottis is iminent and the child needs urgent intubation. Tracheostomy is reserved if the child fails endotracheal intubation.

4. **K**

5. **A**
   Management is similar to that for asthma.

Question 118: Answers

1. **C**
   Sistrunk's operation or thyroglossal cyst excision includes excision of the body of the hyoid bone to prevent recurrence.

2. **F**
   Neck scrofula is treated medically and not surgically.

3. **E**
   Branchial cysts are excised when not in an infected state.

4. **H**
   Total thyroidectomy is offered to a patient with anaplastic thyroid carcinoma, but the prognosis is still poor, and the patient will not survive 6 months.

5. **I**

Excisional biopsy is necessary to exclude malignancy, i.e. squamous cell carcinoma.

Question 119: Answers

1. **D**

Acoustic neuroma is a cerebellopontine angle tumour and causes cranial nerve palsies via direct compression.

2. **H**

Subarachnoid haemorrhage results from a cerebral aneurysm with rebleed peaking at 14 days.

3. **L**

Medulloblastoma occurs in the cerebellum and accounts for the patient's cerebellar signs. It also leads to obstructive hydrocephalus of the fourth ventricle.

4. **G**

A space-occupying lesion in a woman treated for breast carcinoma is most likely due to a cerebral metastasis. However, a metachronous malignancy can also occur.

5. **K**

The classic 'lucid' period following a 'minor' head trauma may obscure the true diagnosis and make light of the gravity of the situation.

Question 120: Answers

1. **L**

Wegener's granulomatosis is confirmed by biopsy of the involved tissue.

2. **G**

Goodpasture's syndrome is confirmed by detecting anti-glomerular basement antibody.

3. **L**

Bronchial carcinoma is suggested by the presence of hypertrophic pulmonary osteoarthropathy and a solitary lung nodule. Tissue biopsy is required for a definitive diagnosis.

4. K

Pulmonary embolism and infarct can present with haemoptysis. The golden standard for diagnosis is pulmonary angiogram.

5. C

Bronchiectasis is suggested here and can be confirmed by bronchography if the patient is stable.

Question 121: Answers

1. A

2. B

3. D

4. L

5. J

Question 122: Answers

1. B

2. G

The groove sign, a depression between the inguinal and femoral nodes, is associated with the nodes in lymphogranuloma venereum caused by *Chlamydia trachomatis* infection.

3. F

Granuloma inguinale is associated with Donovan bodies detected in the edge scrapings.

4. E

H. ducreyi is the organism responsible for chancroid.

5. D

Primary syphilis presents with a solitary primary chancre.

Question 123: Answers

1. **B**
P. *pyocaneus* is the organism behind malignant otitis externa.

2. **H**
B. *burgdorferi* is the organism responsible for Lyme's disease.

3. **J**
E. *coli* is one of the most common organisms associated with spontaneous primary peritonitis.

4. **A**
B. *anthracis* is contracted from contaminated carcasses.

5. **G**
Gas gangrene is associated with C. *perfringens*.

Question 124: Answers

1. **B**
Stein–Leventhal syndrome is the severe form of polycystic ovarian disease.

2. **F**
Kallman's syndrome, an isolated gonadotrophin deficiency, is associated with anosmia and colour-blindness.

3. **A**
Prolactinoma is associated with prolactin levels of at least 2000 mμ/L. Cimetidine is associated with hyperprolactinaemia but not as severe as in this case.

4. **D**

5. **K**

Question 125: Answers

1. **G**
For the diagnosis of gout, serum uric acid is not as specific as joint fluid analysis for negatively birefringent crystals.

2. G
   With pseudogout or calcium pyrophosphate arthropathy the crystals are positively birefringent.

3. D
   Anti-nucleolus antibody is detected in up to 60% of patients with systemic sclerosis.

4. I
   CREST syndrome, a variant of systemic sclerosis is associated with anti-centromere antibody.

5. L
   Primary Sjögren's syndrome is associated with anti-Ro antibody in 70% of cases.

Question 126: Answers

1. A

2. C

3. E

4. K

5. I

Question 127: Answers

1. H

2. C

3. F

4. M
   Traveller's diarrhoea is associated with *E. coli* infection.

5. E

Question 128: Answers

1. K
   Zollinger–Ellison syndrome or gastrinoma is associated with high gastric acid output.

2. A

3. B

4. D
   Familial polyposis and Gardner's syndrome are both risk factors for colorectal carcinoma. These patients often develop carcinoma by the age of 40!

5. E

Question 129: Answers

1. B

2. A

3. C

4. E

5. G
   The presence of the Philadelphia chromosome gives the patient a poor prognosis.

Question 130: Answers

1. B
   Lupus pernio and erythema nodosum are associated skin lesions with sarcoidosis.

2. G
   Lupus vulgaris, a condition resembling 'wolf-gnawed skin', is also referred to as tuberculosis of the skin.

3. **L**
   Granuloma anulare and necrobiosis lipoidica are both associated with diabetes mellitus.

4. **K**
   These fingernail and bed changes are typical of dermatomyositis.

5. **H**
   Eruptive xanthelasmas are associated with either diabetes mellitus or hyperlipidaemia.

Question 131: Answers

1. **E**
   This patient's chief concern will be massive blood loss. No delay should be taken to crossmatch blood. Blood should be transfused immediately. The blood pressure may be misleading, as she is wearing an antishock garment. An external fixator applied by the orthopaedic surgeons will aid in pelvic fracture stabilisation and stem blood loss.

2. **B**
   As both the nasopharynx and oropharynx are compromised, tracheostomy to achieve an airway is essential.

3. **C**
   With *H. influenzae* epiglotittis, endotracheal intubation may be difficult. It is necessary to have an ENT surgeon at hand to perform an emergency tracheostomy if the inflamed epiglottis impedes endotracheal intubation.

4. **C**
   Glandular fever can present as acute airway obstruction. Death from glandular fever occurs from failed endotracheal intubation. It is wise to have an ENT surgeon at hand to perform an emergency tracheostomy if necessary.

5. **J**
   An acute asthmatic attack is treated initially with oxygen and salbutamol. If necessary IV hydrocortisone is added.

Question 132: Answers

1. **B**
   A condom is advisable to prevent acquisition of sexually transmitted diseases but alone has a higher failure rate than the pill for contraception.

2. **A**

3. **A**

4. **C**
   Age over 35, smoking, and varicose veins are all strong contraindications to the oral contraceptive.

5. **J**
   Recent glandular fever or recent acute hepatitis are both contraindications to the oral contraceptive.

Question 133: Answers

1. **H**
   This is injected directly into the uterus. If all else fails, a hysterectomy is required.

2. **F**

3. **E**

4. **D**
   A trial of syntocinon is given before proceeding to a low transverse Caesarian section.

5. **A**

Question 134: Answers

1. **A**

2. **I**

3. C

4. B

5. D

Question 135: Answers

1. C

2. B

3. F

4. I

5. H

Question 136: Answers

1. I

2. C

3. B

4. L
Dysthymia presents in adolescence usually as a result of a major loss in childhood or chronic stress. The depression lasts for at least 2 years.

5. F

Question 137: Answers

1. A
Intrathoracic airway obstruction is either caused by respiratory syncytial virus or by asthma. With a history of other family relations afflicted, bronchiolitis is more likely.

2. D

3. F

4. G
   Chlamydia trachomatis is contracted by the newborn via genitally-infected mothers.

5. B
   Viral croup is most likely. Although epiglottitis should also be considered.

Question 138: Answers

1. B

2. D
   Epileptic fits arise from cerebral calcification.

3. C

4. F
   This is a rare condition occurring from maternal contraction of chickenpox during the first trimester.

5. K

Question 139: Answers

1. A

2. F

3. B

4. D

5. E

Question 140: Answers

1. A

2. C

3. E

4. M

5. G

Question 141: Answers

1. I
   Dysphagia, stridor, dysphonia or an expanding neck haematoma are all indication to explore a penetrating neck wound.

2. H

3. C
   Prompt insertion of a needle or chest tube into the left pleural space is indicated to relieve the pneumothorax.

4. I
   Immediate surgical exploration is warranted. An on-table angiogram can be obtained simultaneously.

5. I
   Traumatic diaphragmatic rupture is associated with deceleration injuries and requires prompt surgical exploration.

Question 142: Answers

1. D
   Posterior shoulder dislocations are associated with seizures.

2. L
   Twisting injuries of the leg are associated with spiral fractures of the tibia.

3. **G**
   Volkmann's ischaemic contracture of the forearm is associated with both brachial artery injury and supracondylar fracture of the humerus.

4. **I**
   Stress fracture of the shaft of the second or third metatarsal bone may not be evident immediately by the person or on X-ray.

5. **E**
   Navicular fracture may not be evident on X-ray initially but the patient should be treated on suspicion.

Question 143: Answers

1. **J**

2. **K**
   Divarication of the rectus abdominis muscles is associated with multiple pregnancies and chronic abdominal distention. The gap is palpable on exam.

3. **I**
   Spontaneous splenic rupture following minor blunt trauma is associated with infectious mononucleosis.

4. **B**
   Bleeding oesophageal varices is often the cause of massive haematemesis in children.

5. **B**

Question 144: Answers

1. **I**

2. **B**
   Ruptured berry aneurysms account for most of the cases of subarachnoid haemorrhage.

3. **E**

4. D

5. L

Question 145: Answers

1. E
Pneumocystis carinii pneumonia is most likely.

2. J

3. K
Carcinoma of the breast with pleural metastases is most likely.

4. G
Although pulmonary embolus or infarct may also be considered.

5. E
Bronchial carcinoma is also in the differential diagnosis.

Question 146: Answers

1. G

2. I

3. J

4. C

5. E

Question 147: Answers

1. B
This is an autosomal dominant inherited condition. The stridor is caused by laryngeal oedema.

2. G
The combination of spiking fevers and spindle-shaped swelling of the finger-joints is suggestive of JRA.

3. **H**

Acute rheumatic fever may present with migratory poly-arthralgia and carditis. This can manifest as a new murmur, in this instance of aortic regurgitation.

4. **K**

Aortic stenosis may give rise to syncope and be mistaken for a seizure.

5. **I**

Question 148: Answers

1. **H**

2. **D**

3. **C**

4. **E**

5. **F**

Question 149: Answers

1. **B**

Colposcopy to further examine the cervix and concomitant cryotherapy should be undertaken. 5-Fluorouracil and excision with diathermy are both treatment options for viral warts.

2. **G**

Ectopic pregnancy should be treated as an emergency.

3. **C**

4. **A**

The patient needs a diagnostic laparoscopy.

5. **F**

Question 150: Answers

1. **A**
   Pica or in this case eating lead paint gives rise to a profound anaemia.

2. **G**

3. **K**
   Opioid withdrawal gives a similar presentation except GI symptoms are of diarrhoea and not nausea and vomiting.

4. **J**

5. **M**
   Thiazide diuretics increase serum lithium levels. This patient is exhibiting signs of lithium toxicity.

Question 151: Answers

1. **A**
   In uncomplicated urinary tract infection, the most common organism is *E. coli*.

2. **E**
   This patient harbours the organism in the vagina.

3. **B**

4. **H**
   P. mirabilis releases ammonia which alkalinises the urine.

5. **C**
   Erysipelas is caused by Group A streptococcus.

Question 152: Answers

1. **F**
   Cefotaxime is the drug of choice for *H. influenzae* epiglottitis.

2. **D**
A single dose of IM or IV gentamicin as prophylaxis is recommended prior to catheterisation.

3. **C**

4. **I**

5. **A**
Clostridium difficile is associated with antibiotic-associated pseudomembranous colitis and is treated with vancomycin.

Question 153: Answers

1. **C**
A CT scan of the head is unnecessary in the absence of signs of increased intracranial pressure. A skull X-ray to look for skull fracture is more than adequate.

2. **D**
Non-accidental injury should be considered here. The history does not fit with the injuries. A chest X-ray to exclude rib fractures is required.

3. **H**
This child is exhibiting signs of increased intracranial pressure with hypertension and bradycardia. For a 2-year-old the resting heart rate should be greater than 95 beats/min. The blood pressure is too high for a 2-year-old.

4. **D**
In a 2-year-old, an AP chest view will more than adequately image the neck and chest to reveal a radioopaque coin lodged in the cricopharyngeal region.

5. **A**
The history is suggestive of autoimmune thrombocytopaenic purpura, which is associated with recurrent epistaxis and easy bruisability. Low platelet count on FBC would lead one to investigate further for platelet antibodies.

Question 154: Answers

1. **H**
   An ABI of less than 0.4 indicates critical ischaemia. Intermittent claudication is indicated by an ABI of between 0.9 and 0.4.

2. **C**
   The lumbar puncture demonstrates high protein content consistent with a viral illness.

3. **J**

4. **F**
   Collapse of the vertebrae from myeloma deposits has led to cord compression.

5. **A**
   This young boy has suffered a MCA infarction secondary to sickle cell anaemia.

Question 155: Answers

1. **B**

2. **B**

3. **A**

4. **B**
   Evidence-based medicine involves using both individual clinical expertise and the best available external evidence to determine patient's care.

5. **A**

6. **B**
   It suggests determining the accuracy of a diagnostic test by finding proper cross-sectional studies of patients harbouring the disorder.

7. **A**

8. A

9. B
It may raise the cost of patient's care also.

10. B

Question 156: Answers

1. C

2. G

3. J

4. I

5. K
The group B streptococcus organism is harboured in the mother's vaginal canal.

Question 157: Answers

1. A
Aminoglycosides impair neuromuscular transmission.

2. B
The ECG changes are consistent with hyperkalaemia. Peak T waves are also seen on ECG.

3. E
Otoxicity is associated with both aminoglycosides and loop diuretics and is more pronounced in elderly patients with renal failure.

4. G
The complications of intestinal bypass surgery include renal stones (hyperoxaluria), metabolic acidosis, and cirrhosis.

5. J
Acute Addisonian crisis is precipitated by abrupt withdrawal of steroids, stress, sepsis, or surgery. This patient may have had steroid-induced hypoadrenalism.

Question 158: Answers

1. **A**
   Malignant hyperthermia may be precipitated by halothane or by succinylcholine.

2. **B**
   Chvostek's sign is a sign of hypocalcaemia which may occur following thyroidectomy and injury to the parathyroid glands.

3. **E**
   Aspiration pneumonia may occur in a patient with post-operative ileus, drowsiness, or with altered swallowing.

4. **I**
   This patient is in urinary retention.

5. **K**
   This patient may need blood replacement.

Question 159: Answers

1. **H**
   Tabes dorsalis is a manifestation of syphilis occurring 10–35 years after primary infection and results from degeneration of the dorsal columns and nerve roots. Argyll Robertson pupils are associated with syphilis.

2. **B**
   Abulia or coma-vigil, contralateral lower limb paresis, and urinary incontinence are all signs associated with the carotid system, i.e. involving the anterior cerebral artery.

3. **A**

4. **D**

5. **E**
   Subacute combined degeneration of the cord is associated with vitamin B_{12} deficiency.

Question 160: Answers

1. **B**

2. **C**
Budd–Chiari syndrome occurs from thrombosis of the major hepatic veins and has been associated with oral contraceptives.

3. **I**
Rupture of a mucocoele appendix can give rise to pseudo-myxoma peritonei.

4. **H**

5. **D**

Question 161: Answers

1. **A**
Children can acquire lead poisoning by eating lead paint chips.

2. **D**

3. **G**
Cyanide is found in many rodenticides and fertilisers and causes poisoning by inhalation or ingestion.

4. **H**
Carbon monoxide poisoning occurs from inadequate venti-lation, in this case from the gas fireplace.

5. **I**
Insecticides contain inhibitors of cholinesterase and lead to the accumulation of acetylcholine.

Question 162: Answers

1. **A**

2. **C**

3. L

4. F

5. H

Question 163: Answers

1. C

2. D

3. A

4. G

5. F

Question 164: Answers

1. A

2. A

3. A
This comes under the heading of corporate accountability.

4. A
This policy is also incorporated in corporate accountability.

5. A
This is a form of an internal mechanism for clinical perform-ance.

6. A
The CHI is one of the two new external bodies.

7. A
The NICE is the other new external body created as an external mechanism.

8. A

9. B

10. B

Question 165: Answers

1. E

2. F

3. A

4. B
Although diagnosis is often missed until adolescence, when lack of secondary sex characteristics is noted.

5. J

Question 166: Answers

1. F

2. E
The Widal test is used to diagnose typhoid fever. However, it is not as reliable as a marrow culture.

3. B
Syphilis is diagnosed by VDRL (Venereal disease laboratory slide test).

4. I
Weil's disease is caused by *Leptospira interrogans*.

5. A
Paul Bunnell or Monospot is used to diagnose glandular fever.

Question 167: Answers

1. H
Diaphragmatic rupture can be diagnosed on chest X-ray by the presence of bowel or the nasogastric tube in the chest.

2. G

This usually arises from chest injury sustained by hitting the steering wheel with great force.

3. C

4. I

Open pneumothorax is treated by covering the wound with a piece of gauze which is taped down along three sides to act as a flutter-valve.

5. D

Kussmaul's sign is a classic sign for cardiac tamponade as is Beck's triad. However, not all patients present with classic signs!

Question 168: Answers

1. K

A Glasgow Coma Scale of 3 is the lowest score possible.

2. J

A GCS of 8 or less or absence of a gag reflex are both indications for intubation.

3. F

No mention of airway management has been made and therefore should be included in the initial assessment of this patient.

4. F

Penetrating objects should be left in situ until surgery. Again airway assessment is always the first priority in management of head injuries.

5. G

Hypotension should not be assumed to be caused by brain injury.

Question 169: Answers

1. C

Acute back strain is treated conservatively.

2. **F**

Night pain and pathological fractures should make one suspicious for underlying pathology.

3. **G**

Acute cauda equina syndrome requires urgent decompression.

4. **D**

Mechanical back pain is treated conservatively.

5. **H**

Intervertebral disc prolapse is the commonest cause of root pain.

Question 170: Answers

1. **B**

Collar and cuff sling should NOT be used. This sling will increase the downward pull on the lateral part of the clavicle.

2. **A**

Collar and cuff slings are used for fractures of the humerus.

3. **C**

Pathological fractures require surgical intervention.

4. **C**

Transverse fractures of long bones are highly suspicious of pathological fractures.

5. **I**

The Gallows traction is used for children under the age of 2.

Question 171: Answers

1. **A**

Battle's sign (bruising over the mastoid process), raccoon eyes (periorbital bruising), haemotympanum, and CSF leak in the ears or nose are all signs associated with basal skull fracture.

2. **F**

3. **E**
Concussion is the transient loss of consciousness without accompanying neurological signs.

4. **H**

5. **C**
If the dura was breached, the diagnosis is one of open skull fracture.

Question 172: Answers

1. **A**

2. **C**
Surgical repair is undertaken in athletes or associated rotator cuff tear injuries.

3. **D**
Painful arc syndrome is treated with injections of local anaesthetic and steroids. The syndrome is due to degenerative changes of the supraspinatus tendon.

4. **A**
Acromio-clavicular joint subluxation or dislocation is treated conservatively with a broad arm sling followed by mobilisation.

5. **G**
The Hippocratic technique is a one-man technique. The Kocher's manoeuvre requires an assistant for counter-traction. Pain may be a limiting factor to successful reduction.

Question 173: Answers

1. **B**
A locked knee is a classic sign of meniscal injury. Haemarthrosis is delayed.

2. **J**
PCL rupture is suggestive with a history of posterior force on the tibia.

3. **K**

The anterior draw test is demonstrated here. Often the joint needs to be explored under general anaesthesia to make a diagnosis, as movement is limited by pain.

4. **E**

Septic arthritis or pus in the joint requires urgent washout and lavage under GA.

5. **I**

Rheumatoid arthritis usually presents as symmetrical poly-arthropathy but may present as monoarticular arthropathy as in this case. Rheumatoid factor is negative in 30–40% of patients.

Question 174: Answers

1. **B**

This is the treatment for hyperglycaemic hyperosmolar non-ketotic coma.

2. **C**

This is the treatment for diabetic ketoacidosis. The anion gap is 38.

3. **E**

Propranolol has been known to induce hypoglycaemia.

4. **G**

This patient is most likely septic from a chest infection.

5. **H**

This patient has probably self-injected her husband's insulin and has factitious hypoglycaemia.

Question 175: Answers

1. **A**

Mallet finger or avulsion of the extensor tendon is treated in a mallet splint.

2. **H**

3. C

A distal lesion at the level of the wrist causes loss of thumb abduction.

4. E

Sensory loss solely on the palm can occur by hitting the heel of the hand against an object with force.

5. I

Ulnar collateral ligament injury of the thumb is also known as gamekeeper's thumb or skier's thumb.

Question 176: Answers

1. F

2. G

3. A

4. B

A bone scan may be necessary to confirm a stress fracture.

5. D

Question 177: Answers

1. E

Cervical strain or whiplash is treated conservatively.

2. B

Jefferson's fracture is managed by 6 weeks in skull traction followed by 6 weeks in a firm cervical collar.

3. A

It is mandatory to visualise the C7/T1 junction to clear a C-spine X-ray.

4. F

5. G
The hangman's fracture is lethal if both pedicles are displaced. Undisplaced fractures are also at risk and require immobilisation for 12 week in a halo-body cast.

Question 178: Answers

1. N
This autoimmune response to a myocardial infarction occurs weeks to months later.

2. C
In this case, infective endocarditis is the cause of the tricuspid regurgitation.

3. G
This is an autosomal dominant inherited condition of inter-ventricular septum hypertrophy.

4. D
Marfan's syndrome is associated with aortic regurgitation.

5. B
Exertional syncope is a symptom of aortic stenosis. The systolic murmur is classically diamond-shaped.

Question 179: Answers

1. B
Fat embolism is associated with long bone fractures.

2. G
Traumatic injury to the liver or bile ducts is suggested.

3. D
Cerebral injuries do not in themselves cause hypotension. Other causes must be excluded.

4. H

5. K

Question 180: Answers

1. **F**
The patient either has a haemothorax or pneumothorax. A chest tube in the 9th ICS will cover both possibilities.

2. **G**

3. **F**

4. **J**

5. **I**
The cause of the EMD includes tension pneumothorax or cardiac tamponade.

Question 181: Answers

1. **A**
Atropine is given to patients with symptomatic bradycardia.

2. **E**
Third-degree AV block is managed with a transvenous pacemaker.

3. **C**

4. **C**
The patient is in ventricular fibrillation.

5. **H**

Question 182: Answers

1. **A**

2. **H**
The ECG shows changes of nonparoxysmal junctional rhythm consistent with digoxin toxicity. This has been precipitated by concomitant verapamil therapy, which is known to increase digoxin levels by 70–100%!

3. **F**

4. **I**
The patient is in cardiogenic shock.

5. **K**
Vagal manouevres may convert the rhythm back to sinus. If not, drug therapy may be necessary.

Question 183: Answers

1. **C**
The patient has coeliac disease.

2. **A**
The patient has developed pseudomembranous colitis, which is treated with vancomycin or metronidazole.

3. **E**
The baby has intussusception. This can be both diagnosed and treated by barium enema.

4. **F**
This baby may have Hirschsprung's disease which is confirmed by rectal biopsy.

5. **G**
This patient most likely has Wilson's disease and should avoid copper-containing foods.

Question 184: Answers

1. **E**

2. **A**
The child most likely has acute epiglottitis. The initial treatment is securing her airway. Here endotracheal tube intubation is warranted.

3. **J**
A silent chest is an ominous sign of life-threatening asthma and requires aggressive management.

4. I

In view of her extensive facial injuries, endotracheal intubation may be impossible.

5. C

The man has airway obstruction secondary to severe glandular fever or acute epiglottitis. In either case, if ETT intubation has failed, urgent cricothyroidotomy is warranted.

Question 185: Answers

1. A

Hypertension will contribute to ongoing epistaxis. Nifedipine is advisable to lower the patient's BP. She will then need to see her GP for regular antihypertensive therapy.

2. K

Any patient on warfarin who presents with epistaxis should have a clotting screen checked. Treatment with vitamin K may be required. However, the haematologist should be consulted for advice if this is the case.

3. F

A food bolus containing bone is at high risk for perforating the oesophagus and needs prompt attention.

4. G

This patient can be managed conservatively at first with buscopan, a muscle antispasmodic. She will need an outpatient barium swallow upon discharge.

5. D

This patient will need a sialogram, if the parotid swelling reoccurs.

Question 186: Answers

1. A

This organism can give rise to necrotising pneumonia when contracted through contaminated ventilators.

2. F

Yersinia enterocolitica mimics acute appendicitis. It can be cultured in the stool.

3. G

4. D
   Clostridium difficile is the organism responsible for gas gangrene.

5. E
   Clostridium perfringens is the organism responsible for pseudo-membranous colitis.

Question 187: Answers

1. A
   A chest X-ray may show air in the soft tissues, but a gastro-graffin swallow is conclusive in the diagnosis of oesophageal perforation.

2. E

3. G
   A technetium scan should be arranged to investigate for Meckel's diverticula.

4. F

5. H

Question 188: Answers

1. A
   The patient has allergic rhinitis, most likely due to dust mites.

2. G
   The patient is clearly reacting to penicillin. Immediate treatment for anaphylaxis is advised.

3. E
   A double-blinded food challenge is more diagnostic for food allergy than RAST or skin testing.

4. H
   Cystic fibrosis may be associated with nasal polyposis.

5. F

This patient may have hereditary angioedema with C1 esterase deficiency. The patient will have measurable C1 levels and a low C4 level.

Question 189: Answers

1. B

This fungal infection needs urgent surgical debridement and IV amphotericin therapy.

2. D

3. C

Although not conclusive without histology, one must be suspicious of lymphoma in any patient with unilateral enlargement of the tonsil.

4. G

5. A

Malignant otitis externa is associated with infection with *Pseudomonas pyocaneus*.

Question 190: Answers

1. F

Hepatic adenoma is demonstrated on CT scan. Because the adenoma is hypervascular, liver biopsy is contraindicated. This tumour is associated with oral contraceptive use.

2. H

This patient is showing signs of Fitz–Hugh–Curtis syndrome or gonococcal peritonitis. Cervical culture will be positive. The RUQ pain is from adhesions.

3. E

This patient has acute cholecystitis. Murphy's sign is RUQ pain worse on inspiration.

4. G

Alcoholic hepatitis is diagnosed by liver biopsy.

5. **A**
This patient has Crohn's disease.

Question 191: Answers

1. **C**

2. **E**

3. **G**
Mefenamic acid is an antiprostaglandin.

4. **H**
Provera is started on day 14 for a 10-day course.

5. **I**
Here hysteroscopy is advised to look for uterine polyps or other pathology.

Question 192: Answers

1. **A**

2. **G**
As her symptoms are not incapacitating, no treatment is required. When she becomes pregnant, she will not be menstruating.

3. **F**

4. **B**
Danazol is an androgen derivative and therefore the patient must be warned of possible hirsutism and acne.

5. **I**
Laparotomy is required to assess for torsion or rupture of the ovarian cyst and remove the affected ovary.

Question 193: Answers

1. **A**
   This requires urgent incision and drainage to prevent a cauliflower ear.

2. **B**
   This was probably the result of an infection with *Pseudomonas pyocaneus* many years earlier.

3. **F**

4. **I**

5. **D**

Question 194: Answers

1. **D**

2. **G**
   This patient is in left heart failure.

3. **H**
   This patient has angina and should be treated initially with GTN and then maintained on nifedipine, a calcium channel blocker. Propranolol is contraindicated, as he is an asthmatic.

4. **B**
   This patient is a candidate for CABG.

5. **A**
   This patient is experiencing a myocardial infarction.

Question 195: Answers

1. **F**
   Medical therapy should be initiated. Mesalazine is a newer aminosalicylate that avoids the side-effects of sulfasalazine.

2. **E**
The liver and spleen are at high risk of injury from blunt trauma to the abdomen.

3. **C**
Acute cholecystitis is managed conservatively until an urgent ultrasound can be arranged.

4. **A**

5. **D**
This patient has toxic megacolon and is at high risk of perforation when the transverse diameter of the colon exceeds 6 cm.

Question 196: Answers

1. **B**
Treatment involves gently squeezing the glans and rolling the foreskin back over.

2. **A**

3. **C**
There are associations with dialysis, sickle cell anaemia, and pelvic malignancy.

4. **E**
There are associations with Riedel's thyroiditis and with Dupuytren's contracture.

5. **H**
Impotence may be a complication of AAA repair and of radical prostatectomy.

Question 197: Answers

1. **F**

2. **C**

3. **B**

4. **M**

5. **K**